FASCIA UNLEASHED

Optimize Performance and Prevent Injuries with this Cutting-Edge Therapy

Copyright © 2024
Vanessa A. Gibson

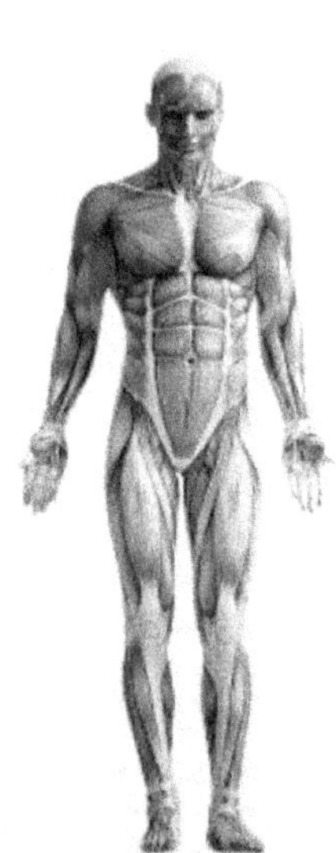

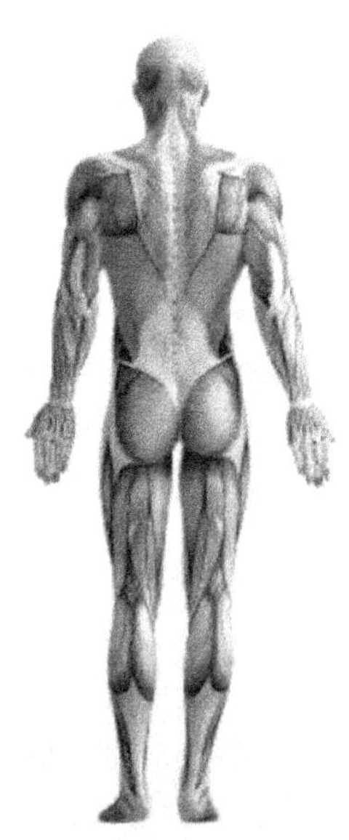

TABLE OF CONTENTS

Introduction

Welcome to Fascia Unleashed, a journey that delves into the complex fabric of your body's connective tissue and goes beyond the confines of traditional treatment. As a therapist who is passionate about improving human performance and avoiding injuries, I cordially encourage you to learn more about the cutting-edge treatment that is described in these pages.

The mysterious fascia, a network of connective tissues often overshadowed by its more obviously visible cousins, muscles, and joints, is at the center of our investigation. But rather than being a passive observer, fascia plays a crucial role in the symphony of physical movement by providing the structural support required for ideal function.

Together, we will explore the secrets of fascia, including its structure, variety of layers, and significant impact on our mobility, stability, and general health. Gaining an understanding of fascia is essential to opening up new possibilities for enhancing physical performance.

This treatment, which goes by the moniker "Unleash the Power of Fascia," was born out of a combination of biomechanical know-how and scientific investigation. This technique, which was created by a group of experts committed to expanding the realm of conventional medicines, is firmly rooted in evidence-based procedures.

In this book, we will explore the history of the treatment, looking at the painstaking research that formed its foundation and the process of development that brought it to where it is now. As a therapist, I promise to provide you with more than simply a routine of exercises—I'll give you a thorough grasp of the biomechanics and scientific basis of each approach.

We shall go further into the therapy itself in these chapters, including its methods, applications, and the practice of self-treatment. In contrast to traditional treatments that concentrate only on joints and muscles, "Unleash the Power of Fascia" focuses on the fascial network, which is often disregarded. This treatment is a harmonic fusion of research and practice that is intended to change your path toward improved physical well-being.

My mission as a therapist is to empower you by providing you with a comprehensive plan for your physical health. We will talk about how, at any fitness level, this treatment fits in perfectly with your current training regimen. The ideas presented here provide a complete answer for everyone, whether they a professional athletes aiming for maximum performance or a person recuperating from physical illnesses.

Come discover with me the advantages of "Unleash the Power of Fascia"—better performance, more flexibility, fewer injuries, and faster recovery. This therapy is a dynamic addition to your normal training routine rather than a stand-alone treatment.

You may be confident that the methods in this book have been thoroughly tried by therapists, fitness specialists, and athletes alike, in addition to being the result of considerable scientific study. Our team's unrelenting dedication is to continuously develop these methods so that you obtain the most recent, evidence-based treatments.

Get ready to go on a life-changing adventure. "Unleash the Power of Fascia" is a concept that aims to help you realize the full potential of your body, not merely a treatment. My job as a therapist is to support you as you go through this investigation and provide you with the information and resources you need to maximize your potential and avoid harm.

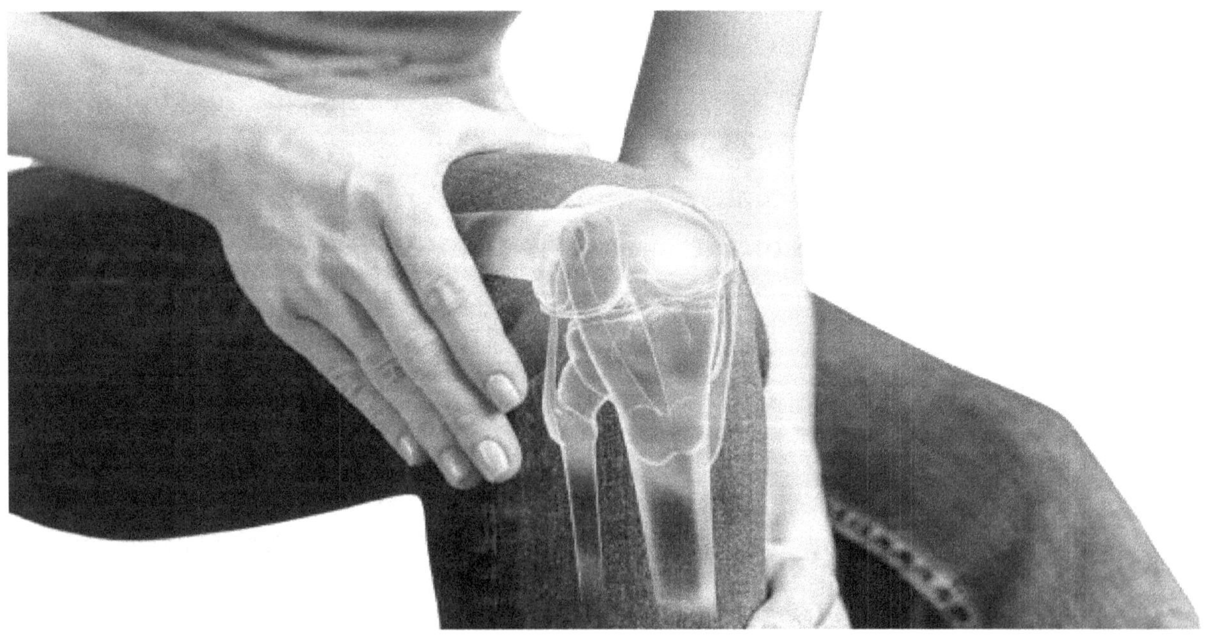

Understanding Fascia

Fascia appears in the rich story of human anatomy as a quiet conductor that deftly navigates the geography of the body. Understanding fascia means taking a deep dive into the often-ignored field of connective genius.

The entire body is constructed from fascia, a network of fibrous tissues that are intricately interwoven. Its structure is more complex than the simple outlines of muscles and bones; instead, it is a three-dimensional, continuous matrix that surrounds, holds up, and links every internal component. Imagine it as the supple yet strong threads that weave movement, stability, and structural integrity into a tapestry.

Understanding the layers of fascia is like learning the secret language of the body. Every layer of fascia, from the deep fascia surrounding muscles to the superficial fascia just under the skin, contributes differently to preserving the delicate balance necessary for ideal function. Within this complex structure, fascia affects every action we make by giving muscles the tension and flexibility they need to operate together smoothly.

However, its impact goes beyond the field of mechanics. Fascia plays an active role in the dynamic symphony of biological processes, not just a passive one. Fascia is a sensory organ that transmits crucial information about the location and state of the body. Its receptors are rich in information that contributes to our kinesthetic awareness, even beyond its involvement in movement.

Recognizing fascia's profound effects on general health requires understanding it. Disproportions or imbalances in this network of connective tissue might appear as restricted mobility, weakened joint health, or even be a factor in persistent pain. Understanding the complexities of fascia helps us to realize the body's full potential for resilience and peak performance.

We will explore the composition, function, and essential role that fascia plays in the dance of movement as we work through the secrets of fascia in the pages ahead. Get ready for an enlightening adventure as we explore the transforming potential of fascia for improved physical well-being and learn how to read its language.

Definition and Composition

Fascia is an unsung hero in the complex world of human anatomy, where every fiber and sinew plays a part in the beautiful choreography of movement. Fascia is a thin but ubiquitous network of connective tissues. Understanding fascia's fundamental concept and composition—which serve as the cornerstones of its significance—is necessary before we can begin a thorough investigation of the subject.

The term "fascia," which comes from the Latin word meaning "band" or "bandage," refers to the dynamic, continuous network of collagenous fibers that permeates the whole body. It is a living matrix that not only surrounds and supports bones, muscles, and organs but also weaves them together in a symphony of interconnection, making it a structural wonder. Fundamentally, fascia is the quiet maestro directing the dance of physical motion.

In conventional anatomical discourse, this architectural matrix is often disregarded, although it is crucial to our comprehension of biomechanics and physical functioning. Fascia is more than just a covering; it is a flexible, responsive structure that is essential for dispersing tension, conveying force, and preserving the body's structural integrity.

Fascia's complex makeup is what gives it its greatest adaptability. Fascia is made up mostly of collagen, the most prevalent protein in the human body, and together they form a tapestry that is resilient and strong. Collagen fibers arrange themselves in a variety of ways to meet the unique requirements of distinct anatomical locations.

Another crucial ingredient that gives fascial tissues their suppleness is elastin. This adds to the dynamic responsiveness needed for smooth movement by enabling fascia to resist strain as well as to rebound. The ground material lubricates and allows collagen and elastin fibers to glide smoothly between fascial layers. It is a gel-like matrix.

This mosaic of ground material, elastin, and collagen creates a dynamic continuum that can adjust to the particular needs of various tissues and locations. A greater understanding of fascial composition's function in preserving structural integrity and promoting mobility emerges as we peel back the layers.

Fascia is a dynamic system that adapts to the demands made on it, far from being a static covering. Fascia dynamically remodels itself in response to external stimuli, movement patterns, and postures via complex cellular communication. Its dynamic character emphasizes how important it is for maintaining body structures as well as affecting the fluidity and efficiency of movement.

We will go further into the layers of fascial anatomy and examine the subtle differences in composition across various body locations in the next chapters. A deeper comprehension of fascia's function in the complex dance of human movement will emerge from this investigation, setting the stage for the groundbreaking treatment that you will find in the pages that follow.

Get ready to explore the fascinating realm of fascia, where composition and definition come together to create the story of our physical existence.

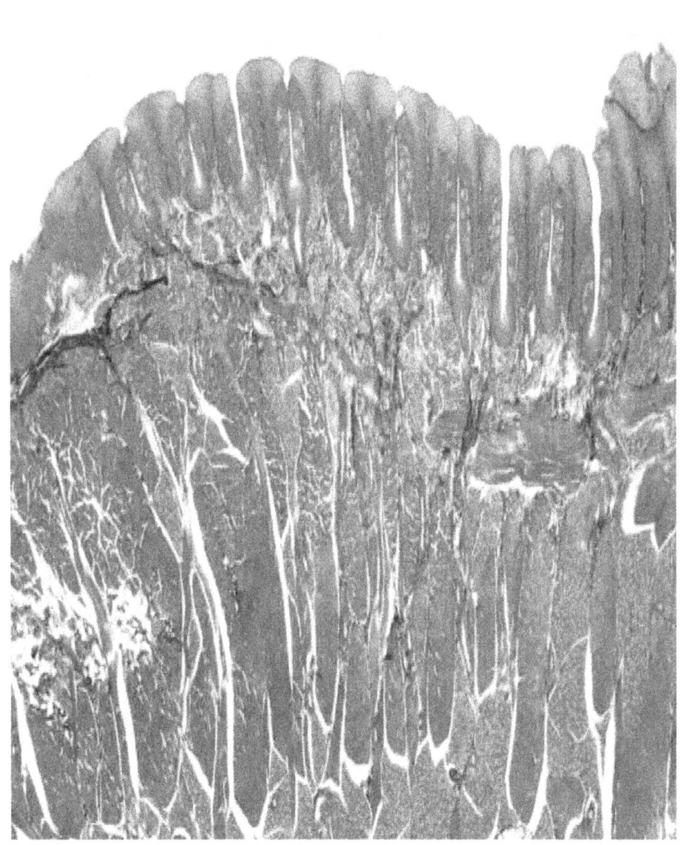 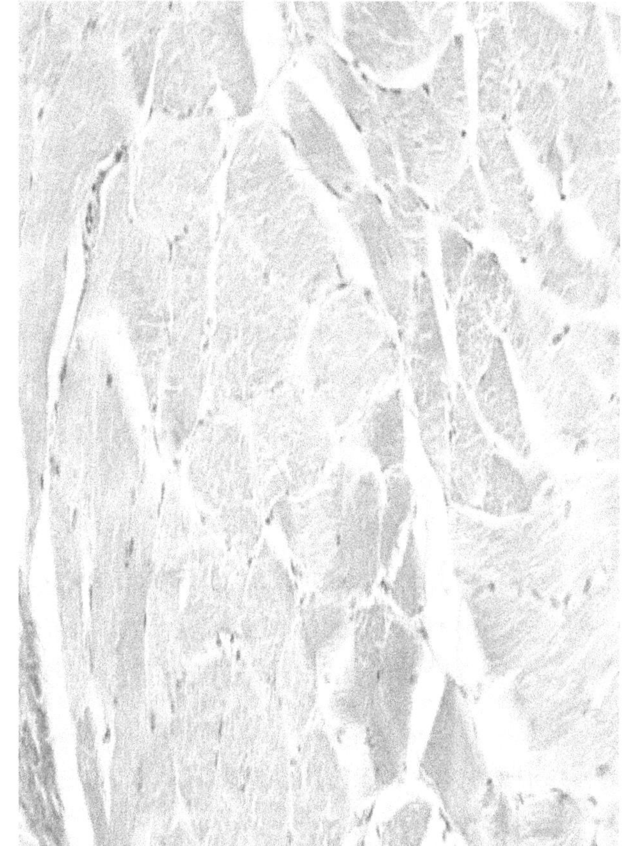

The Role of Fascia in Body Movement

Salutations to everyone who desires health and vigor. Let us go out on a thoughtful voyage today, a tour that reveals the complex fascia tapestry, the silent orchestrator behind every action we make.

Fascia is an unsung hero in the field of bodily mobility; it creates a complex web that encloses and affects every muscle, joint, and organ. Think of it as your body's architectural blueprint—a living, breathing structure that molds your physical experience.

The nuances of fascia frequently provide me comfort in my work as a therapist. It serves as the unifying factor that combines dissimilar parts to create a smooth, well-coordinated dance. Imagine a dance, where the hands of fascia, which are unseen to the naked eye, guide every elegant and flowing movement. It is the steadier, unseen force that guarantees your motions are both elegant and meaningful.

Think about how easy it is to raise your arm. Your muscles carry out the activity, while the fascia facilitates, supports, and permits a fine range of motion. Fascia is a dynamic conductor that changes its tension and flexibility in reaction to each movement you make, not simply a passive structure.

Let's now consider flexibility, a property that is often connected to the suppleness of muscles. However, what dictates how expansive your motions are is the state of your fascia. Your body can adjust to the many demands of life with elegance when it has a robust and well-nourished fascial network.

Within the therapeutic context, we recognize the body's delicate messages. Fascia is a communicator as well as a structural component. Your nervous system receives crucial information from fascia via a network of sensory receptors woven across its layers. Your brain receives information on the location and state of every bodily part from this silent conversation.

As a therapist, I am aware that the body is a vessel that holds the echoes of emotional events rather than just a physical object. Because fascia can hold stress, it becomes a storehouse for both emotional and physical impressions. We start a journey of release and renewal for the body and soul by attending to the health of your fascial network.

Think of fascia in this therapeutic investigation as an essential component of your overall health rather than as a separate entity. Fostering harmony between mind and body may be achieved by nourishing and comprehending your fascial environment. It is evidence of how your emotional and bodily identities are intertwined.

Importance of Fascial Health in Athletic Performance

When it comes to sports accomplishment, strength of muscles, cardiovascular endurance, and technique mastery are often highlighted. The complex network of connective tissues that permeates the body, known as the fascia, is a crucial but usually disregarded member of this performing ensemble.

Basic Assistance for Flowing Motion

Fundamentally, the fascia offers a structural base that is necessary for the performance of dynamic motions. Imagine it as the structural foundation that not only preserves the health of our musculoskeletal system but also makes it easier for us to coordinate in a way that allows us to play our best sports.

Improving Elasticity for Motion Without Effort

The capacity of fascia to provide the muscles flexibility is one of its most important functions. Athletes can perform moves with more fluidity and accuracy because of this elasticity, which also improves their range of motion and flexibility. During physical activity, a well-conditioned fascial network stores and releases energy effectively, much like a natural spring.

Syncing and Integrated Kinetic Chains

In the kinetic chain, fascia acts as a unifying factor to ensure that muscles, joints, and tendons work in harmony. For exact, coordinated motions, such as an explosive start in a run, a complex routine in gymnastics, or quick direction changes in basketball, this integration is essential.

Adaptability to Injuries

Keeping your fascia in peak condition is a preventative step against injuries. Athletes may drastically lower their risk of common injuries like strains, sprains, and tears by treating imbalances, limitations, or adhesions within the fascial network. Forces applied during physical activity are absorbed and distributed by a robust fascial structure, which serves as a protective shield.

It's critical for athletes who want to exceed their performance limits to comprehend the function of fascia. Muscle function is supported by a robust fascial network, which increases power output. For individuals aiming to reach their absolute athletic potential, this means having more speed, agility, and efficient force generation.

A holistic approach to sports training is essentially introduced by placing a high priority on fascial health. It recognizes the interconnectivity of the body's tissues, going beyond the traditional emphasis on specific muscles and joints. Fascial conditioning is a paradigm shift toward thorough physical preparation that may be included in training programs.

It is impossible to exaggerate how crucial fascial health is for athletes who want to excel in their particular sports. It is an essential part of a comprehensive, performance-driven strategy, not just an extra factor. Acknowledging the importance of fascial health promotes adaptability, productivity, and a basis for long-term athletic success.

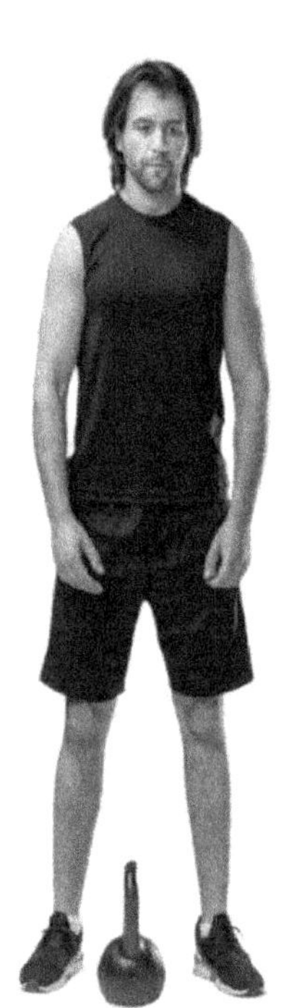
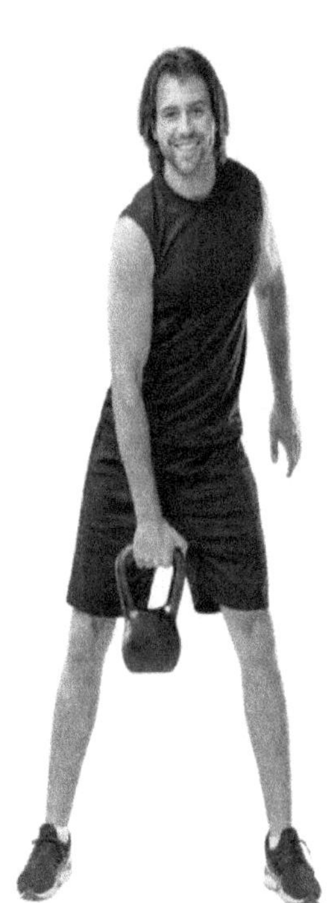
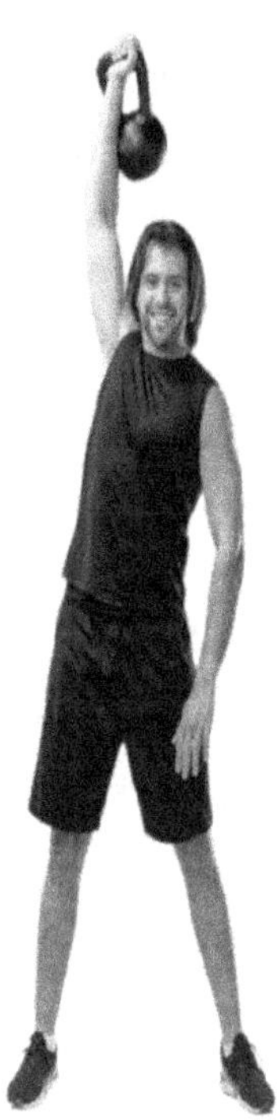

Chapter 1

THE FASCIAL NETWORK

Anatomy of the Fascial System

Any sheath, sheet, or other dissectible mass of tissue that joins, envelops, or divides the body's deep structures is referred to as fascia.

Generally speaking, fascia comes in two varieties:

- cutaneous fascia
- profound fascia

The connective tissue that divides the skin from the underlying muscle tissue is referred to as the superficial fascia (also known as tela subcutaneous, hypodermis, and subcutaneous tissue).

Deep under the skin and subcutaneous tissue is the thick, well-organized connective tissue known as the deep fascia. It envelops the viscera, muscles, and other tissues. There are several kinds of deep fascia, depending on where it is located. Among them are:

muscle fasciae (also known as fasciae musculorum)

Body cavity fasciae (also known as fascia cavitated trance)

The primary role of the fasciae is to support and shield the body's deep organs and tissues. Furthermore, fasciae transfer movement from muscles to bones, reduce friction between muscles and sometimes act as the site of attachment for skeletal muscles.

Layers and Types of Fascia

The fascial system is represented by a wide range of layers in the complex structure of the human body, each of which plays a distinct role in maintaining the organism's overall structural integrity and functioning. To clarify the unique traits and functions of the many layers and forms of fascia, this section attempts to disentangle their complexity.

The Interface Between Skin and Deeper Structures is Known as Superficial Fascia.

The superficial fascia is a layer that is just below the skin's surface. This fascial layer, which consists of loose connective tissue and houses adipose tissue, blood vessels, and nerve endings, is essential for thermoregulation. In addition to its structural role, superficial fascia supports the gliding motions between the skin and underlying tissues and acts as a channel for lymphatic drainage.

Deep Fascia: Embracing Organs, Muscles, and More

The deeper fascia, a thicker, more robust layer that surrounds muscles, nerves, and organs, is located underneath the superficial fascia. Deep fascia provides structural support and compartmentalization by encircling muscle groups in sheaths. It performs the functional role of transmitting force, enabling coordinated motions, and preserving the spatial connections between anatomical parts.

Internal Organ Nurturing and Protection by Visceral Fascia

The visceral fascia extends farther into the body to envelop internal organs in a supporting and shielding embrace. This layer helps the organs move around and operate properly in addition to acting as a structure for them. The delicate balance between organ movement and structural stability inside the visceral cavity is maintained in large part by visceral fascia.

Parietal Fascia: Linking the Skeletal Structure to the Muscles

The contact between the skeletal structure and deep fascia is formed by parietal fascia. It gives muscles a membrane coating that helps to transmit mechanical forces during muscular contractions and anchors the muscles to the bones. Coordinated movement and joint stability are greatly dependent on the parietal fascia's capacity to preserve the spatial connections between muscles and bones.

Fascial Networks in Muscles: Endomysium, Perimysium, and Epimysium

Different layers of fascia further refine their responsibilities at the microcosmic level, within the individual muscles. The whole muscle is covered with the epimysium, which acts as a protective coating. The perimysium divides the muscle into fascicles by extending inside, and the endomysium envelops each muscle fiber to create a microenvironment that is necessary for force transmission and nutrition exchange.

Comprehending the many strata and varieties of fascia reveals the complex organizational concepts that oversee the body's connective tissue system. With its properties and roles, each layer synergistically adds to the fascial system's overall harmony and functioning. This sophisticated understanding paves the way for an in-depth investigation of therapeutic measures intended to maximize fascial health and, therefore, improve human function.

Fascial Connections in the Body

The idea of fascial linkages is a testimony to the smooth integration of different anatomical components within the complex fabric of the human body. The complex web of connective tissues that makes up the fascial system is interrelated and extends much beyond isolated areas. Understanding the comprehensive influence of this network on body function and biomechanics requires an understanding of the vast nature of fascial linkages.

1. The Meaning and Character of Facial Connectivity

The fascial system is continuous and linked, which leads to the formation of fascial linkages. Individual fascial compartments do not exist in isolation; rather, they interact and communicate with neighboring areas to build a complete network that spans the whole body. A constant tensional framework is created by this dynamic interaction, allowing for coordinated movement and support across a variety of anatomical systems.

2. Surface to Substantial Associations

On the outside, the fascial connections appear as layers covering the muscles, giving them a structural base. This includes the superficial fascia that lies just below the skin's surface and serves as a cohesive interface between the muscle below and the body's outer layer. Further in, the fascial strands entwine themselves with ligaments, tendons, and muscle fibers to form a smooth continuity that spans organ systems and joints.

3. Correlates with Biomechanics

Fascial connections have a crucial role in mediating biomechanical coordination, which highlights their relevance. The fascial network transfers forces and tensions throughout the body during muscle contraction and joint articulation, resulting in a kinetic chain reaction. Because of the interconnectedness of this biomechanics, energy can be transferred efficiently and muscles may perform harmoniously, resulting in ideal movement patterns.

4. Proprioception and Facial Connections

Fascial connections are essential for proprioception, the body's sense of its location in space, even outside of its biomechanical function. Feedback about tension, strain, and pressure is provided by sensory receptors located in the fascial matrix, which affects the nervous system's regulation of muscle contractions and joint stability. Maintaining postural stability and improving movement precision depend on this proprioceptive feedback loop.

5. Effect on Integration of Functions

Facial connections affect whole functional units in addition to individual muscles. The longitudinal channels that connect distant anatomical areas are known as myofascial meridians, and they are facilitated by the connections between the superficial and deep layers of fascia. Professionals working in the movement disciplines, rehabilitation, and sports performance need to understand these relationships because they provide a more comprehensive approach to training and injury prevention.

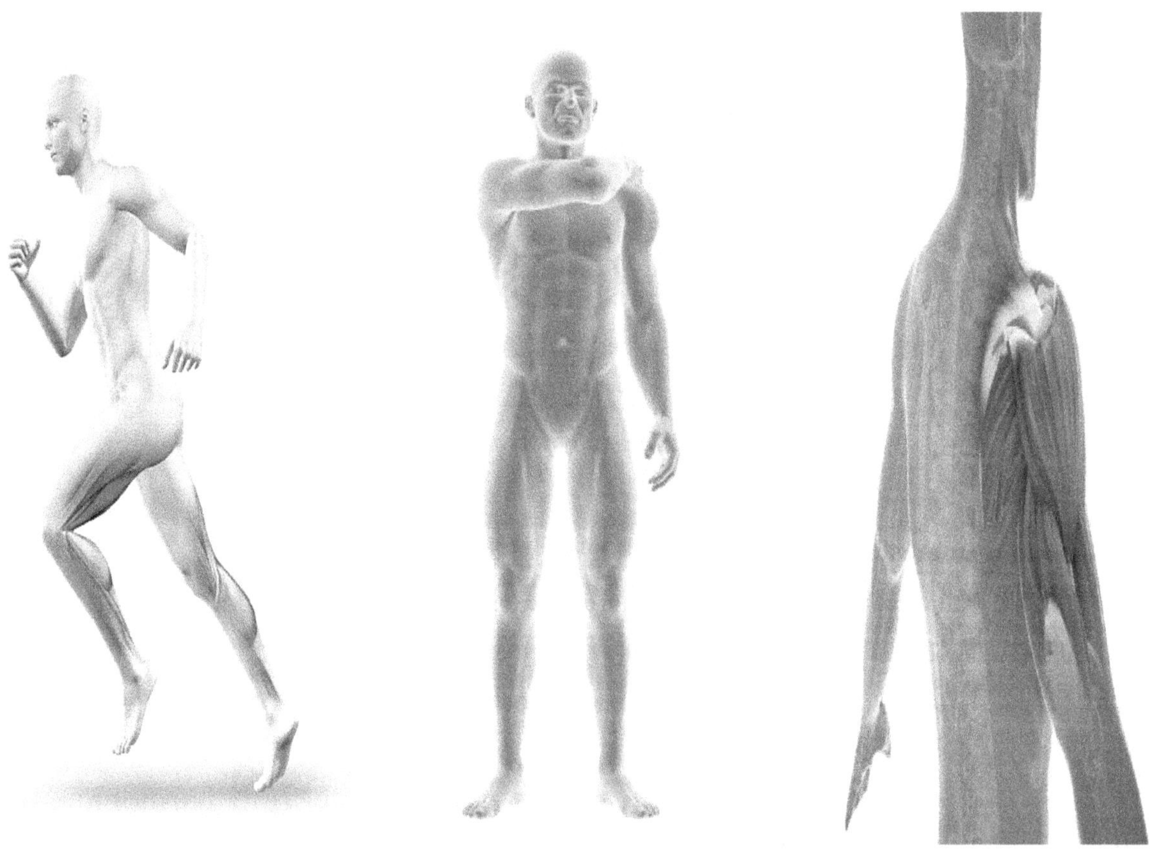

The fact that fascia has such a strong effect on movement patterns is evidence of its function as a dynamic, interwoven web that runs throughout the whole body. Fascia is portrayed as a passive structural element, but in reality, it plays a crucial role in organizing, maximizing, and forming movement. This thorough investigation explores the many ways that fascia profoundly affects patterns of movement.

1. Constant Tensional Network: An Anatomical Structure

Fundamentally, fascia encloses muscles, tendons, ligaments, and even bones in a continuous tensional network. This networked matrix functions as a biomechanical structure that transfers forces produced during motion. Tensional forces within the fascial system are distributed across different anatomical components when muscles contract and joints articulate. A synergy is produced by this dynamic interaction, enabling efficient and well-coordinated movement patterns.

2. Force Transfer: The Kinetic Chain Effect

An essential function of fascia is to transmit the forces produced by contractions of muscles. Rather than restricting motion to certain muscles or joints, the fascial system enables a kinetic chain reaction. Forces applied to one area of the body easily spread across the fascial network, impacting other areas. The cohesion and fluidity of movement patterns are facilitated by this coordinated transfer of forces.

3. Myofascial Meridians: Extended Connectivity Pathways

The idea of myofascial meridians is one prominent example of how fascia affects movement. These are far-off anatomical locations connected by longitudinal channels of fascial connection. Knowing about myofascial meridians is essential to understanding how changes in one area of the body may affect the whole system. An example of the interconnectedness of movement patterns is how a limitation in the lower back fascia may affect shoulder mobility.

4. Accurate Movement and Proprioception

The body's capacity to sense its location in space, or proprioception, is facilitated by the abundance of sensory receptors found in fascia. These sensors react to variations in the fascial matrix's pressure, stretch, and tension. These proprioceptive signals provide input that affects how the nervous system regulates posture, joint stability, and muscle contractions. This complex interaction is essential for improving movement accuracy and adjusting to changing conditions.

5. Plasticity and Adaptability: Changing Reactions to Movement

Fascia has a great degree of flexibility and adaptability in response to patterns of movement. Fascia modifies and adapts its structure in response to external stimuli via mechanisms such as mechanotransduction, which is the process by which mechanical forces impact cellular responses. The fascial system can accommodate a broad variety of movement patterns, from complex, precise movements to strong, dynamic activities, thanks to its versatility.

6. Effect on Dynamics of Posture

Fascia sustains the musculoskeletal system's alignment and provides support, which plays a major role in postural dynamics. The body's stability in both static and dynamic postures is influenced by the fascial connections that exist between muscles and across joints. The efficient execution of coordinated actions and the maintenance of an upright posture are contingent upon the fascial system's ideal balance.

To sum up, the way fascia affects movement patterns is a result of a complex and multifaceted interaction between biomechanics, connection, and adaptation. This knowledge goes beyond conventional theories about the musculoskeletal system and emphasizes the crucial part fascia plays in arranging the intricate patterns of human movement. Understanding the subtleties of fascial influence helps us better understand how improving fascial health may enhance movement quality, athletic performance, and general well-being.

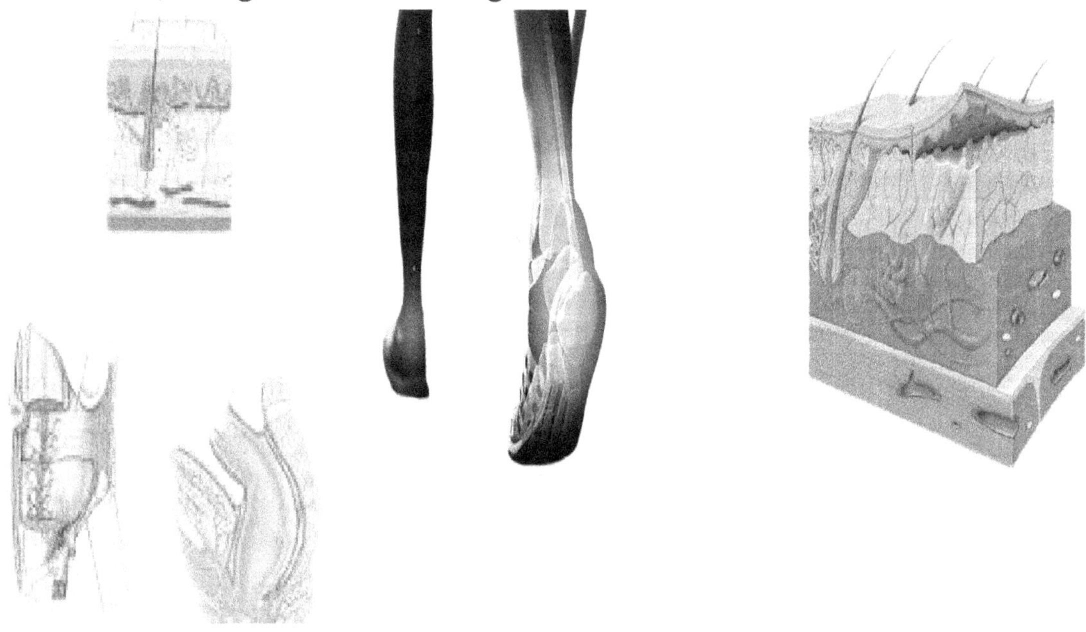

Chapter 2

UNVEILING THE THERAPY

Origins of "Unleash the Power of Fascia"

"Unleash the Power of Fascia" has its origins in a scientific investigation that goes beyond traditional therapy methods. Experts with extensive backgrounds in fascial fitness, biomechanics, and evidence-based research collaborated to develop this ground-breaking treatment. One may characterize the path that resulted in the creation of this revolutionary treatment as nothing less than a scientific adventure.

1. Growth and Change

The narrative starts with everyone realizing how complex fascia is to the human body. In contrast to conventional treatment approaches that prioritized muscles and joints, the creators of "Unleash the Power of Fascia" set out to solve the secrets of the often disregarded fascial network. It became clear that a treatment aimed at restoring fascia's optimal health and function might completely change the way we think about physical health.

The creation of the treatment included a combination of biomechanical knowledge, anatomical insights, and a profound respect for fascia's plasticity. As the treatment developed, it took cues from emerging research and scientific discoveries that highlighted the critical role fascia plays in regulating mobility, strength, and general physiological balance.

2. The Therapy's Biological Basis

A thorough grasp of the biomechanics driving fascial dynamics is fundamental to the genesis of "Unleash the Power of Fascia". The treatment is a carefully planned intervention meant to function in harmony with the body's inherent biomechanics rather than just a set of exercises. This biomechanical understanding guarantees that every method used in the treatment is intentional, focused, and in line with the intrinsic characteristics of fascial tissues.

The designers of the treatment realized that the best outcomes could only be obtained by incorporating a thorough understanding of fascial biomechanics into the therapeutic strategy. By doing this, they paved the way for a treatment that actively improves the fascial network's general resilience and health in addition to addressing current problems.

3. Research and Scientific Foundations

There's a strong scientific basis for "Unleash the Power of Fascia". The treatment is the outcome of thorough investigation and scientific testing, not a hypothesis or anecdotal evidence. Through systematic investigations, researchers, physicians, and practitioners worked together to confirm the therapy's effectiveness and make sure its tenets meet the strictest criteria of scientific examination.

The roots of the treatment are entwined with an emphasis on evidence-based practice, guaranteeing that each method and procedure is founded on accepted scientific knowledge. This commitment to study serves to both validate the therapy's legitimacy and present it as a dynamic, ever-evolving method that is sensitive to new scientific discoveries.

When we explore the history of "Unleash the Power of Fascia," we see how scientific curiosity, biomechanical know-how, and a dedication to improving human performance come together. This treatment offers evidence of the possibility of revolutionary discoveries under the direction of a strict scientific methodology. Its continuous progress is fueled by an unwavering quest to comprehend and optimize the complex network of fascial connections that supports our physical existence.

Development and Evolution

The path toward a transformational approach to fascial wellbeing is a paradigm change in our understanding of and approach to optimizing the complex network of connective tissues that make up the human body. This growth is a dynamic process that integrates scientific research, creative thinking, and a dedication to holistic well-being rather than a linear path.

1. Understanding the Significance of Fascia

This evolutionary strategy was born out of a deep understanding of the importance of fascia. The dynamic and diverse quality of this connective tissue was recognized by pioneers in fascial health, beyond its conventional position as a passive structural element. It became clear that therapeutic approaches may be redefined by gaining a greater comprehension of the function of fascia in mobility, support, and general physiological equilibrium.

During this first stage, practitioners and researchers broke with traditional thinking by exploring the scientific subtleties of fascial anatomy, biomechanics, and the body's integrative function.

2. Combining Anatomical Knowledge

This paradigm-shifting technique required careful integration of anatomical knowledge throughout development. With the development of imaging technology, a more complete picture of the structure and interconnection of fascia emerged, offering hitherto unattainable insights into the workings of complex fascial networks. The tenets and methods of the treatment were developed on this fundamental understanding.

An appreciation of the intricacy of the fascial system was ingrained along with the therapeutic approach via the integration of anatomical concepts. Understanding fascia as a living, breathing tissue created the foundation for a strategy that addresses the underlying causes of problems with fascial health rather than just treating symptoms.

3. Knowledge of Biomechanics

A thorough biomechanical knowledge of how fascia affects movement patterns and general physiological function is at the core of this evolutionary journey. The treatment was designed to be a comprehensive intervention that works with the body's inherent biomechanics rather than a set of discrete exercises.

During this stage, therapeutic applications and biomechanical concepts were combined to make sure that every method in the approach respected the intrinsic qualities of fascial tissues while still being successful. Here, the progression is typified by a move away from general therapies and toward a focused, individualized strategy that takes into account each person's biomechanical profile.

4. Empirical Investigation and Ongoing Improvement

This paradigm's growth and development in fascial health went beyond theoretical frameworks. A crucial role was performed by meticulous empirical testing and clinical observation. The treatment was continuously improved based on practitioner feedback, real-world results, and ideas from a variety of case studies.

This dedication to empirical testing is indicative of a dynamic and flexible methodology that is sensitive to the rapidly accumulating body of knowledge in a variety of disciplines, from rehabilitation sciences to anatomy. The treatment is continually improving because it is open to new scientific discoveries, advances in technology, and changing demands of people who want better financial health.

The Biomechanics Behind the Therapy

The treatment method is fundamentally a complex dance between science and the body's natural biomechanics. Gaining an appreciation for the subtle and intentional nature of the therapies intended to maximize fascial health requires an understanding of the biomechanics behind the therapy. This investigation explores the scientific foundations that support the effectiveness of the treatment and its compatibility with the unique biomechanical characteristics of the human body.

1. Dynamic Face Tension: The Basis for Motion

An essential component of the biomechanical basis of the treatment is the understanding of fascia as a dynamic tensional network. Muscles, bones, and organs are encircled by a continuous network of connective tissues that affect movement patterns and maintain structural integrity. The therapy strategies are carefully crafted to take advantage of and intensify this natural tension in the fascial system.

It is essential to comprehend the dynamic nature of fascial stress. The therapy's methods make use of the fascial network's capacity to transfer forces during muscle contraction and joint articulation, promoting coordinated movement and enhancing the effectiveness of biomechanical processes.

2. Targeted Release and Stretching: Enhancing Fascial Elasticity

A key component of the therapeutic approach is the use of stretching and releasing methods that are influenced by biomechanics. The treatment acknowledges that the collagenous and elastic components of fascia react dynamically to mechanical stimuli. Targeted stretching seeks to increase fascial elasticity in addition to flexibility.

The treatment aims to maximize the fascial system's elasticity and tensile strength balance by using biomechanically sound concepts. This technique is a precision-guided strategy that is customized to each person's unique biomechanical profile rather than a general stretching program.

3. Coordinated Movement Patterns-Myofascial Chains

Biomechanical knowledge includes myofascial chains, which are fascial connection routes that run the length of the body and link individual muscle groups. The treatment recognizes that these myofascial links arrange movement as a synchronized symphony. Through the treatment of fascial health within these chains, the synergistic functioning of muscles and joints is optimized.

With this biomechanical viewpoint, the emphasis is shifted from discrete treatments to a comprehensive strategy that takes the body's fascial network's interconnection into account. Methods are carefully crafted to affect whole myofascial chains, encouraging balanced movement patterns.

4. Adaptability and Load Distribution: Strengthening Resilience

The therapy's focus on load distribution and fascial system adaptation is guided by biomechanics. The treatment acknowledges that promoting adaptation to a range of movement demands in addition to regulating external stresses is necessary for good fascial health. Methods are intended to improve the fascial system's capacity to disperse stresses uniformly, therefore mitigating localized stress and bolstering systemic resilience.

The idea of mechanotransduction, or the biological reaction to mechanical stimuli, is included in this biomechanical adaptability. The goal of the treatment is to encourage remodeling and improve the fascial tissues' ability to resist and adjust to dynamic biomechanical demands by encouraging positive adaptations within them.

5. Combining Biomechanical Understandings: A Tailored Method

The therapy's dedication to an individualized approach is fundamental to its biomechanical foundations. Understanding that every person has their biomechanical signature, the treatment customizes interventions to meet individual requirements. This tailored method guarantees the accurate application of biomechanical principles that take into account individual differences in anatomy, movement patterns, and lifestyle circumstances.

The therapy's biomechanics are a mix of scientific precision and a profound understanding of the nuances of human movement. Therapeutic procedures are deliberate uses of biomechanical concepts intended to maximize fascial health; they are not random. Through a process that respects the body's inherent biomechanics, the treatment provides a path toward improved mobility, flexibility, and general well-being.

The principles of optimum fascial well-being are based on a strong body of research with continuous studies as support. The therapeutic method is a dynamic system formed by evidence-based principles rather than an arbitrary collection of therapies. This investigation explores the scientific foundations that support the treatment and demonstrates its dedication to the best research practices and ongoing improvement.

1. Evidence-Based Procedures

The therapy's scientific basis is evidence-based procedures that have been painstakingly developed through extensive study. To combine information from anatomical research, clinical observations, and empirical investigations, researchers, practitioners, and clinicians work together. This joint endeavor guarantees that the treatment method is grounded on scientific data, enhancing its legitimacy and efficacy.

Following evidence-based guidelines puts the treatment at the forefront of fascial research developments. This dedication goes beyond conventional treatment approaches, enabling a more flexible and dynamic method of treating the intricacies of fascial health.

2. Extensive Empirical Research

Thorough empirical testing reinforces the scientific basis of the treatment. Methods and procedures are methodically assessed in real-life situations, providing important information about their effectiveness, security, and usefulness. By testing and improving the therapeutic method iteratively, it is ensured that it will continue to be sensitive to the various requirements and subtleties of people seeking financial well-being.

Practical results and theoretical knowledge are connected via empirical testing. It strengthens the therapy's status as a cutting-edge and adaptable modality by enabling it to change in response to new problems, a range of patient profiles, and discoveries in science.

3. Combining anatomy and biomechanics

The combination of anatomy and biomechanics is a fundamental aspect of the therapy's scientific basis. It is essential to comprehend the complex interactions that exist between anatomical variances, biomechanical concepts, and fascial structures. The treatment bases its interventions on the most recent findings in these domains, guaranteeing that every method is anatomically correct and biomechanically sound.

This integration enables the treatment to target the underlying biomechanical abnormalities causing fascial difficulties in addition to the symptoms. Through the use of scientific information to inform treatments, the therapy provides a thorough and focused method for promoting fascial health.

4. Dedication to Continual Investigation

The therapy's focus on continuous research serves as an example of its commitment to scientific excellence. The therapeutic method is always evolving along with scientific understanding. Researchers associated with the treatment do ongoing research, adding to the growing corpus of information on biomechanics, therapeutic methods, and fascial health.

This dedication to continuing research guarantees that the treatment will always be at the forefront of research-based medicine. Furthermore, it makes it easier for new scientific discoveries to be included in the treatment plan, making it more flexible and current in the ever-changing field of science.

5. Cooperation with the Scientific Community

One of the main components of the therapy's scientific basis is collaboration with the larger scientific community. The treatment maintains its connection to fascial scientific developments via establishing collaborations with scientists, organizations, and specialists in relevant domains. This collaborative mentality fosters a culture of continuous growth, information sharing, and increased credibility for the treatment.

 The therapy's scientific basis and supporting studies reflect a dedication to quality, flexibility, and ongoing improvement. Through adherence to the most recent evidence-based procedures and participation in continuous research endeavors, the treatment guarantees that its tenets stay at the forefront of scientific comprehension, providing people with a dependable and state-of-the-art method for boosting fascial well-being.

The Techniques

The methods for optimizing fascial health are carefully devised and are at the heart of the therapeutic approach. These methods combine evidence-based tactics, exact anatomical knowledge, and biomechanical concepts. Every technique is specifically designed to address the complexities of the fascial network, demonstrating a dedication to accuracy and creativity in the search for improved health.

1. Specific and Targeted Myofascial Release

One of the most important techniques is myofascial release, which involves precise and focused manipulation of the fascial tissues. By applying pressure with their hands and stretches, practitioners want to release tension, increase suppleness, and encourage the best possible fascial mobility. The method takes into account the fact that the fascial system is not the same for every person and customizes treatments to target specific adhesion and tension patterns.

The therapy's emphasis on myofascial release recognizes the significance of resolving fascial constraints at their root, which enhances movement patterns and promotes overall structural harmony.

2. Fascial Stretching: Increasing Range of Motion and Elasticity

Techniques for stretching the fascia dynamically contribute to the therapeutic repertory by focusing on improving the suppleness and range of motion of the fascia. This method uses stretching procedures that are individually customized and biomechanically sound, acknowledging the interrelated nature of fascial planes.

Using purposeful and regulated stretching, practitioners seek to maximize the fascial system's adaptability, promoting enhanced flexibility, decreased rigidity, and an increased potential for dynamic movement.

3. Techniques for Tensional Balance: Aligning Myofascial Chains

The body's myofascial chains are interrelated, and this is addressed via tension-balancing treatments. Through the identification and correction of tension and load distribution abnormalities, the goal of these treatments is to bring the fascial system back into balance. Through the alignment of myofascial chains, practitioners want to encourage more efficient and well-coordinated movement patterns.

This method demonstrates a novel strategy that goes beyond localized therapies by acknowledging the influence of fascial connection on overall biomechanical function and its holistic character.

4. Exercises at Home and Self-Care: Empowering People

A major focus of the treatment is equipping clients with at-home exercises and self-care skills. Acknowledging that achieving optimum fascial well-being involves more than just treatment sessions, people are given the resources and techniques they need to go on their path at home. Exercises that are simple yet effective and based on biomechanical principles allow people to take an active role in their health.

This method encourages people to incorporate fascial health practices into their everyday routines for long-lasting benefits by fostering a feeling of agency and self-efficacy.

5. Creative Proprioceptive Education: Enhancing Movement Sequences

Through the use of cutting-edge proprioceptive training methods, the treatment improves body awareness and control, which refines movement patterns. Proprioceptive exercises increase balance, coordination, and neuromuscular control by stimulating the body's proprioceptors in the fascial system.

This method emphasizes the therapy's dedication to a thorough and gradual approach to maximizing fascial health in addition to enhancing other therapies.

6. Combining Mind-Body Techniques for Holistic Health

The treatment incorporates mind-body approaches in addition to strictly physical ones. Breathwork, relaxation methods, and mindfulness all support the patient's overall health and well-being. This integration encourages a balanced and harmonious approach to financial well-being by acknowledging the interconnectedness of mental and physical health.

The methods used in the therapeutic approach are an innovative blend of accuracy. These methods, which are based on biomechanical concepts, anatomical knowledge, and evidence-based tactics, come together to provide a versatile arsenal for maximizing fascial health. Every technique is both a therapeutic intervention and evidence of the therapy's dedication to providing each person with a personalized and practical route toward improved well-being.

Overview of Therapy Sessions

Treatment sessions that are conducted within the concept of enhancing fascial wellness provide a thorough and individualized path to improved physical health and well-being. These meticulously planned sessions include a variety of methods, approaches, and instructional elements, resulting in a comprehensive strategy to address the complex subtleties of the fascial system. An informative synopsis of what to anticipate from these sessions of transformational treatment is provided below:

1. First Evaluation: Comprehending Personal Requirements

Every therapeutic journey starts with a comprehensive first evaluation. Practitioners investigate the patient's lifestyle, movement patterns, medical history, and any particular fascial health issues. The cornerstone for customizing treatment sessions to each patient's specific needs and objectives is this thorough examination.

2. Biomechanical Profiling: Recognizing Trends and Disproportions

In therapeutic sessions, biomechanical profiling is a crucial component. Practitioners locate stress points in the fascial system as well as movement patterns and postural abnormalities by closely observing and evaluating patients. The creation of a customized treatment plan is influenced by this profile, which guarantees that therapies are focused and in line with the person's biomechanical signature.

3. Specific Interventions: Stretching Methods and Myofascial Release

Treatment sessions include specific techniques intended to maximize fascial health. The goal of myofascial release treatments, which include stretching and physical pressure, is to improve fascial mobility and relieve limitations. Improved fascial system flexibility and range of motion are facilitated by customized stretching treatments. With accuracy, these therapies target the distinct patterns found in the biomechanical profile.

4. Tensional Exercises for Balance and Coordination: Body Harmonization

Exercises for coordination and tensional balance are essential components of therapeutic sessions. The goals of these therapies are to lessen asymmetries, encourage harmonic movement patterns, and bring the myofascial chains back to homeostasis. Through the manipulation of the fascial system, these workouts enhance the coordination and efficacy of biomechanical function.

5. Proprioceptive Training: Increasing Awareness of the Body

Novel proprioceptive training is integrated to improve neuromuscular control and body awareness. These workouts sharpen movement patterns and enhance balance and coordination by taxing the fascial system's proprioceptors. Therapy sessions get a dynamic and progressive element from proprioceptive training, which strengthens the connection between the body and mind.

6. Patient Education: Strengthening Practices of Self-Care

An essential component of treatment sessions is education. By providing a greater grasp of biomechanics, fascial health, and the value of self-care techniques, practitioners empower people. Patients are given advice on exercises they may do at home, self-care methods, and lifestyle changes that can help them maintain their well-being outside of treatment sessions.

7. Mind-Body Unification: Encouraging Comprehensive Health

Mind-body techniques are integrated into therapy sessions to support holistic well-being. The sessions include breathwork, mindfulness, and relaxation methods to improve the whole experience. By acknowledging the relationship between mental and physical health, this holistic approach promotes harmony and balance.

8. Progressive Adaptations: Changing in Step with Personal Development

The strategies change as patients go through therapy sessions to meet their evolving requirements. Frequent evaluations and continuous dialogue between clinicians and patients guarantee that the treatment modifications are according to each patient's development, promoting a flexible and adaptable method of maximizing fascial health.

Treatment sessions that are conducted to enhance fascial well-being provide a complex and unique experience. Through the integration of focused treatments, biomechanical understandings, and an all-encompassing viewpoint, these sessions offer people a profoundly transformational experience to maximize their fascial system's potential and cultivate an elevated sense of well-being.

Detailed Techniques for Targeting Specific Areas

It is essential to provide a sophisticated grasp of methods that target certain fascial system regions. Based on anatomical accuracy and biomechanics, these meticulous methods seek to optimize fascial health overall while addressing specific issues. For practitioners looking to improve their skill set in certain areas, here is an instructive guide:

1. Shoulder and neck myofascial release:

Method: Pin and Stretch

- Tell the client to let go of the neck muscles while you gently push on the trigger spots that have been discovered.
- Apply pressure in conjunction with deliberate neck motions, including lateral flexion or rotation, to facilitate the release of tension within the fascial layers.
- Depending on the client's input and the tissue's reaction, gradually raise or reduce the pressure.

Advantages:

- releases tension in the shoulders and neck.
- increases the neck's range of motion.
- increases shoulder and neck suppleness overall.

2. Lower Back Fascial Stretching:

Method: Supine Lumbar Flexion Extension

- Help the client to bend their knees while lying on their back.

- While keeping the client's spine neutral, gently stretch their hips and knees toward their chest.
- To improve lower back fascial release and relaxation, emphasize regulated breathing.

Advantages:
- eases the lumbar fascia's strain.
- improves the lower back's range of motion and flexibility.
- relieves lower back pain for those who experience it.

3. Hip Tensional Balancing Techniques:

Method: Resistance-Induced Hip Abduction and Adduction
- Place the client on their side, with their upper leg elevated.
- Assist the client in performing controlled hip abduction and adduction by adding resistance to the exercise.
- To guarantee that fascial components are activated in a balanced manner, emphasize using the whole hip complex.

Advantages:
- encourages harmony in the tension in the hip fascia.
- improves hip flexion strength and coordination.
- focuses on the imbalances that cause hip pain.

4. Training the Ankles and Feet with Proprioceptive Awareness:

Method: Hand Towel Pulls

- Give the customer a little towel to crumple up with their toes on the floor.
- Promote a deliberate, unhurried motion while highlighting the activation of the intrinsic foot muscles.
- Increase the resistance gradually by using things like a thicker towel or toe spread exercises.

Advantages:

+ enhances the feet's proprioception and balance.
+ strengthens the foot's intrinsic muscles.
+ focuses on problems with ankle instability and plantar fasciitis.

5. Forearm Myofascial Release Technique:

Technique: Compression of the forearm

+ Assist the client in positioning their forearm on a stable surface.
+ Gently compress the whole length of the forearm using your hands, your forearms, or special instruments.
+ To further aid in the release of fascial tension, encourage the client to actively move their wrists and fingers during compression.

Advantages:

+ releases the forearm fascia's stress.
+ helps treat or avoid ailments including carpal tunnel syndrome and tennis elbow.
+ increases the general mobility and flexibility of the forearm.

6. Stretching the Hamstrings with Fascia:

Method: Rotation and Seated Hamstring Stretch

+ Sit the client with one leg straight out in front of them and the other bent, with the foot pressed up on their inner thigh.
+ Tell them to reach for their toes and twist their upper body in the direction of the outstretched leg.
+ Stress the importance of keeping your spine straight and using the fascial structures in your leg's back.

Advantages:

+ targets the hamstrings' fascial limitations.

- enhances range of motion and flexibility for hamstring stretches performed while sitting.
- relieves hamstring tightness in those who have it.
-

Include the Following Teaching Suggestions:

- Throughout the session, give the client's comfort priority and maintain good communication.
- Adjust technique pressure and intensity in response to specific client input.
- To improve proprioception and engagement of the targeted fascial regions, encourage your clients to actively participate in movements.
- Stress how crucial it is to breathe deliberately to maximize the benefits of the methods and encourage calm.

By sharing these specific methods and encouraging a deep comprehension of their uses, practitioners may improve their capacity to target certain areas of concern, which will lead to a more accurate and efficient method of maximizing fascial wellbeing.

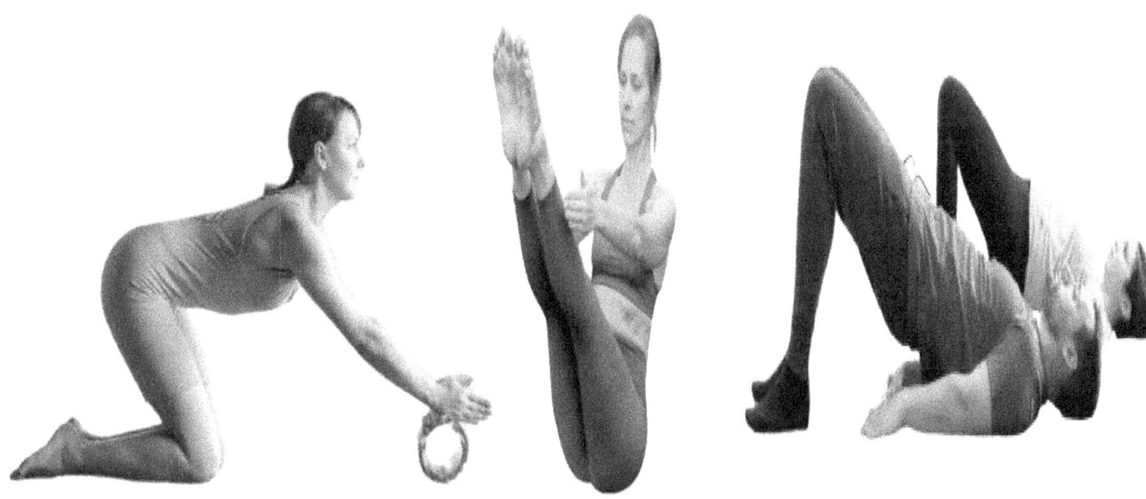

1. Shoulder and neck self-myofascial release:

Tools required: A foam roller or a tennis ball

- Against a wall, comfortably sit or stand with the selected equipment.
- Position the foam roller or ball between the wall and the desired location, such as the shoulders or neck.
- Lean into the device and move it along the targeted muscles to provide little pressure.
- To enable the pressure to loosen financial constraints, pause in intense places.
- Apply pressure and rotate your neck in controlled ways, making little tilts or rotations to achieve a full release.

2. Lower Back Fascial Stretching:

An exercise mat is required as equipment.

- With your feet flat on the mat and your knees bent, lie on your back.
- Grasping one knee with both hands, bring it close to the chest.
- Breathe deliberately so that your lower back may expand and relax.
- To make sure both sides are stretched, switch legs and do the stretch again.
- For long-lasting effects, do this regularly while extending the length progressively.

3. Hip Tensional Balancing Techniques:

Tools required: Band of resistance

- Attach the resistance band's one end firmly to a stationary object.

- With the foot on the other side closer to the anchor point, wrap the band around one ankle.
- Controlled side leg lifts against resistance are achieved by contracting the hip muscles.
- To encourage balance in the hip fascia, pay close attention to maintaining tension throughout the exercise.
- Turn over and carry out the practice again.

4. Training the Ankles and Feet with Proprioceptive Awareness:

Tools required: little towel

- Step barefoot onto a tiny towel that has been placed on the floor.
- Lift your foot arches by utilizing your toes to crunch and hold the towel.
- After a few seconds, release the scrunch after holding it.
- Increase the intensity progressively as you do the workout ten to fifteen times.
- Include toe-spreading exercises by elevating and spreading your toes briskly.

5. Forearm Self-Myofascial Release Technique:

Tools required: A massage ball or a tennis ball

- Put the ball on a level surface while you are comfortably seated.
- Place your forearm over the ball and gently push down.
- Targeting tense spots on the forearm, roll the ball along it.
- To address various fascial angles during the release, rotate your forearm.
- Regularly work on both forearms, particularly if you're feeling sore from doing repeated things.

6. Stretching the Hamstrings with Fascia:

Required equipment: towel or yoga strap

- With one leg straight and the other bowed, take a seat on the floor.
- Using both hands, loop the strap around the foot's sole that has been expanded.
- Maintaining a straight back, bend forward at the hips.
- Along the rear of the outstretched leg, feel the stretch.
- Breathe deeply while holding the stretch for 20 to 30 seconds, then swap sides.

Overarching Guidance for Self-Medication:

- **The Secret Is Consistency:** For cumulative effects, include self-treatment strategies regularly.
- **Listen to Your Body:** Be aware of the cues your body gives you, and change the intensity appropriately.
- **Breath Awareness:** To improve relaxation and the methods' efficacy, engage in deliberate breathing exercises.
- **Adjust as Necessary:** Adjust the methods to suit your comfort level and any prevailing medical issues.
- Drink plenty of water to help maintain the hydration and pliability of fascial tissues.

Individuals may actively optimize their fascia well-being, cultivate flexibility, reduce stress, and enhance their general physical well-being by adhering to these comprehensive self-treatment protocols.

Chapter 4

INTEGRATING FASCIAL FITNESS INTO YOUR ROUTINE

Setting off on a path to maximize fascial fitness requires a deliberate blending of specific workouts, conscious motions, and lifestyle choices. You may unleash the potential for better flexibility, better movement patterns, and general well-being by adding fascial training to your regimen. This comprehensive manual offers a step-by-step plan for incorporating fascial training into your everyday routine:

1. Comprehending Fascial Fitness: The Basis for Overall Health

To maximize the health and performance of the fascial system—a dynamic network of connective tissues throughout the body—specific exercises and motions are a part of facial fitness.

2. Morning Routine for Mobilization: Awaken Your Fascia

Parts:

- ❖ Dynamic Stretching: To stimulate the fascial system and increase blood flow, do mild, dynamic stretches.
- ❖ Foam Rolling: To release tension and improve fascial mobility, use a foam roller for your bigger muscle groups.
- ❖ Breathwork: To improve oxygenation and promote relaxation, use conscious breathing.

Advantages:

- ❖ With more vigor and movement, greet the day.
- ❖ Improve blood flow and lessen rigidity.
- ❖ Set a good example for attentive movement all day long.

3. Take Breaks for Facial Stretching to Add Movement to Your Day

Parts:

- ❖ Micro-breaks: Throughout the day, take brief pauses to do fast fascial stretches.

- Dynamic motions: To activate different fascial lines, including motions like ankle rolls, hip circles, and arm circles.
- Mindful Posture Checks: To avoid fascial constraints, check and correct your posture regularly.

Advantages:

- Combat extended periods of sitting or standing still.
- enhance blood flow and lower the chance of stiffness.
- Develop an awareness of your body and a conscious relationship with your facial system.

4. Focused Fascial Exercises: Weekly Meetings for All-Around Health

Parts:
- Myofascial Release: Apply specific myofascial release methods or implement equipment such as massage balls and foam rollers.
- Stretching exercises that target distinct fascial lines should be included in your regimen.
- Incorporate multi-muscle group workouts into your strength training regimen to enhance integrated fascial conditioning.

Advantages:
- Enhance tissue elasticity and release fascial limitations.
- Develop your strength in a manner that keeps your fascia intact.
- Improve the general quality of your movements and functional fitness.

5. Mind-Body Techniques: Comprehensive Health for Your Fascial System

Parts:
- Practices that stress conscious movement and stretching, such as yoga or pilates, may help to promote fascial health.
- Develop a meditation routine that lowers stress and promotes a healthy mind-body connection.

❖ Breathwork Sessions: Set aside time for concentrated breathing techniques to improve relaxation and oxygenation.

Advantages:
❖ Decrease stress, as it may be a factor in fascial tension.
❖ Encourage a mind-body connection that is beneficial to general health.
❖ Increase mobility and flexibility by moving purposefully.

6. Lifestyle Points to Take into Account: Providing Internal Nutrition to Your Fascial System

Parts:
❖ Hydration: To promote the hydration and pliability of fascial tissues, maintain appropriate hydration.
❖ Nutrient-Rich Diet: To promote fascial health, give priority to foods high in collagen, antioxidants, and other vital nutrients.
❖ Adequate Rest: To encourage tissue regeneration and repair, make sure you get enough sleep and rest periods.

Advantages:
❖ Encourage the fascial tissues' flexibility and resiliency.
❖ Improve your connective tissues' general health from a holistic standpoint.
❖ Encourage the best possible healing and regrowth.

7. Monitoring Your Progress: Examining Your Journey Towards Facial Fitness

Parts:
❖ Movement Journal: Document all of your everyday physical activities, workouts, and any changes in your body's sensations.
❖ Flexibility Evaluations: Monitor your progress by regularly evaluating your range of motion and flexibility.
❖ Feedback Mechanisms: Monitor your body's reaction to various workouts and modify your regimen as necessary.

Advantages:
❖ Remain inspired by praising your accomplishments.
❖ Determine any trends or locations that could need further care.

- ❖ Develop a greater understanding of how your body reacts to fascial fitness exercises.

8. Seeking Expert Advice: Collaborating with Specialists

Parts:

- ❖ Consultation with a Fascial Fitness Professional: You may want to look for advice from a licensed therapist or fascial fitness teacher.
- ❖ Workshops and seminars: To enhance your knowledge and hone your skills, enroll in specialized seminars or workshops.
- ❖ Cooperation with Healthcare Providers: To guarantee a comprehensive approach to your well-being, engage in communication with healthcare providers.

Advantages:

- ❖ Get tailored advice based on your particular requirements.
- ❖ Gain access to professional expertise to maximize the benefits of your fascial exercise regimen.
- ❖ Make sure that a customized and safe strategy is used to handle certain issues.

You may use these elements in your regimen to create a dynamic, all-encompassing approach to fascial conditioning. Achieving optimum well-being may be sustained and transformed by combining fascial fitness via focused workouts, mindful movements, or lifestyle choices.

Adopting a comprehensive strategy that takes into account lifestyle, mental, and emotional aspects in addition to physical fitness is necessary to achieve physical well-being. The following doable tactics may be included in your everyday routine for a thorough and all-encompassing approach to physical well-being:

1. Practices of Mindful Movement:

Include:
- Yoga and Tai Chi: These forms of exercise integrate breathing, movement, and awareness to enhance balance, flexibility, and mental clarity.
- Daily Stretching Routine: To increase flexibility and relieve stress, set aside a few minutes each day for stretching activities.

Advantages:
- increases the range of motion and flexibility of the body.
- encourages mindfulness, which lowers stress and improves mental health.

2. Well-Composed Exercise Program:

Add:
- Cardiovascular Exercises: To improve heart health, take up exercises like cycling, swimming, running, or walking.
- Strength Training: Use resistance training to increase muscle mass and boost your metabolism.
- Adaptability and Mobility Workouts: Incorporate movements aimed at improving general flexibility and joint mobility.

Advantages:
- enhances cardiovascular well-being.
- strengthens and facilitates mobility functionally.
- improves general physical stamina and health.

3. Hydration and Nutrition:

Put into practice:

- A balanced diet should consist of a range of foods high in nutrients, such as fruits, vegetables, lean meats, and whole grains.
- Sufficient Hydration: To sustain healthy physical functioning and promote general well-being, sip water throughout the day.

Advantages:

- provide vital nutrients for optimum body functioning and vitality.
- promotes a healthy metabolism and digestive system.
- improves general health and vigor.

4. Restful Sleep:

Ascertain:

- Maintain a Regular Sleep Schedule: Try to get seven to nine hours of good sleep each night.
- Establish a relaxing habit before going to bed, such as reading or doing some light stretching.

Advantages:

- promotes the healing and regeneration of the body.
- improves emotional stability and cognitive performance.

5. Stress Reduction Methods:

Include:

- Practice mindfulness meditation to foster calmness and lower stress levels.
- Exercises for Deep Breathing: To trigger the body's relaxation response, practice deep, diaphragmatic breathing.

Advantages:

- lowers stress-related chemicals and improves cognitive function.
- enhances general well-being and emotional resiliency.

6. Social Networks:

Develop:

- Establish meaningful ties with friends, family, and the community.

＋ Frequent Social Activities: To strengthen a feeling of belonging, take part in social gatherings and activities.

Advantages:
＋ lessens feelings of loneliness and promotes emotional health.
＋ increases life satisfaction and general pleasure.

7. Frequent Medical Exams:

Set priorities:
＋ Normative Health Examinations: Plan routine tests and check-ups for your health.
＋ Consultation with Medical Specialists: Consult a physician about any health issues.

Advantages:
＋ Early identification and management of any health problems.
＋ guarantees a proactive strategy for preserving physical health.

8. Harmony between work and life:

Ascertain:
＋ Establish Boundaries: Clearly state where your personal and professional lives overlap.
＋ Make self-care a priority by setting aside time for enjoyable and calming pursuits.

Advantages:
＋ lowers work-related stress and burnout.
＋ increases general contentment and pleasure with life.

9. Ongoing Education and Development:

Participate:
＋ Opportunities for Learning: Engage in mentally stimulating activities, such as reading, attending classes, or picking up a new skill.
＋ Personal Development: To continue growing, set, and achieve personal objectives.

Advantages:

✛ enhances cognitive function and mental acuity.

✛ encourages a feeling of purpose and achievement.

Using these useful techniques results in a comprehensive and synergistic approach to physical well-being. Taking into account the interdependence of mental, emotional, and physical health opens the door to long-term general well-being in your day-to-day activities.

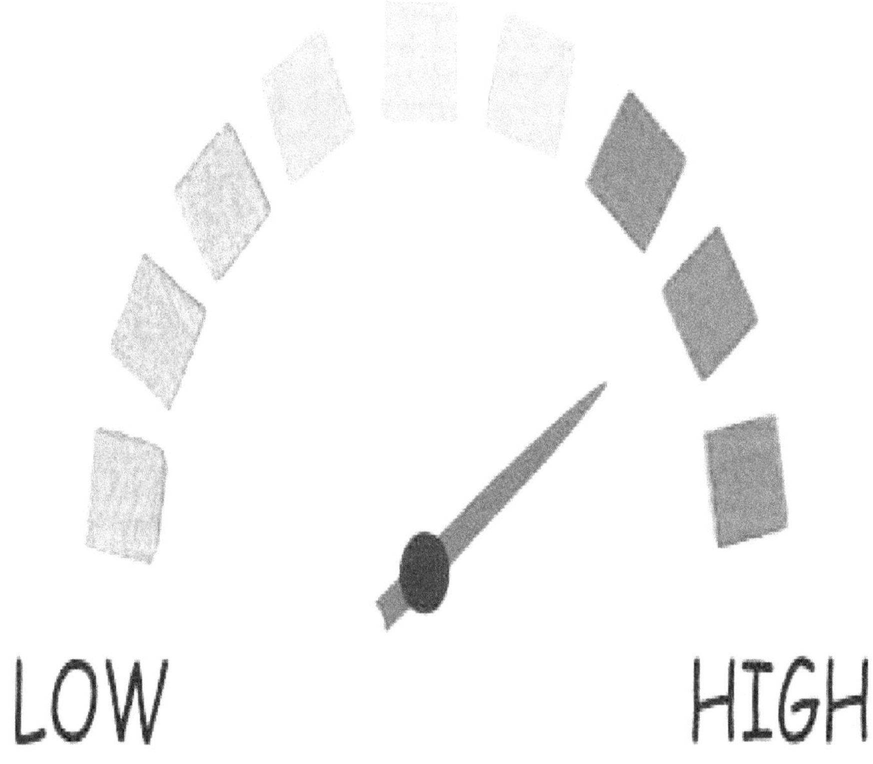

Fostering a feeling of accessibility, empowerment, and long-term success requires designing a fitness or wellness program that is inclusive and adaptable for people of all fitness levels. The following are guidelines for creating and executing a program that accepts participants of all fitness levels:

1. Tailored Exercise Programs:

- Different Intensity Levels: Create training programs that offer a range of intensity levels so that people may choose a degree of difficulty that best fits their level of fitness.
- Exercise adaptations should be made to account for different degrees of fitness. This guarantees that persons with varying levels of experience may engage in the activity with assurance.

Advantages:
- accommodates people with varying levels of fitness abeginning.
- encourages people to feel successful on many levels.

2. Increasing Difficulties:

- Gradual Progression: Allow participants to advance at their speed by introducing a progressive increase in complexity or intensity over time.
- Periodic evaluations: Include periodic evaluations to monitor each person's development and establish new goals in response to their progress.

Advantages:
- urges people to think more positively by setting attainable goals.
- honors significant anniversaries and personal accomplishments.

3. Effective Communication:

+ Transparent Instructions: Make sure that participants grasp the correct form and technique by giving them clear, succinct instructions for each activity.
+ Encouragement: To inspire people and create a welcoming and friendly atmosphere, use language that is upbeat and supportive.

Advantages:
+ lessens fear and creates a friendly environment.
+ encourages people to take part with confidence.

4. A Variety of Exercise Choices:

+ Variety of Activities: To accommodate a variety of tastes and interests, provide a varied selection of workouts and activities.
+ Provide cross-training alternatives so that individuals may choose exercises based on their interests and fitness objectives.

Advantages:
+ attracts a wider range of people with different interests in fitness.
+ gives freedom to choose workouts that fit individual objectives.

5. Knowledgeable Teachers:

+ Trained to Adapt: Make sure that instructors have received the necessary training to modify exercises to accommodate students of varying fitness levels.
+ Educators use inclusive language, recognizing and honoring a range of skills.

Advantages:
+ fosters a secure and encouraging atmosphere.
+ Increases participant trust in the advice given.

Improving your current training routine entails carefully incorporating additional components that work in concert with your present program. Athletes, fitness enthusiasts, and people on wellness journeys may all benefit from carefully combining different training modalities to reach new heights in terms of performance, recuperation, and general well-being. Here's how you include extra elements for maximum effect smoothly:

1. Determine the Training Goals:
- Present Objectives: Make sure you understand your main goals for performance or fitness.
- Opportunities for Development: Determine which particular areas of your training need more attention.

- Combines complementing elements in a way that is tailored to your overall objectives.
- Guarantees a focused and calculated approach to integration.

2. Combine Flexibility and Mobility:

- Prioritize active warm-ups before your primary exercises to improve joint mobility and flexibility.
- Dedicated Mobility Sessions: To address any restrictions found, set aside certain sessions for focused mobility exercises.
- enhances flexibility and joint health, which lowers the chance of accidents.
- increases the range of motion and overall quality of movement.

3. Recuperation Techniques:
- Active Recovery Days: Include low-impact exercises like swimming or walking to increase circulation without significantly raising stress levels.
- Rehabilitation Techniques: To speed up muscle healing, look at methods like foam rolling, massages, and contrast baths.

- speeds up the healing process in between hard training sessions.
- lowers tiredness and soreness in the muscles.

4. Nutritional Assistance:

- Strategic Supplementation: Take into account supplements that support your training requirements, including electrolytes for hydration or protein for muscle repair.
- Balanced Nutrition: Make sure your daily food intake meets your energy needs and your fitness objectives.

- maximizes recuperation and performance with specific dietary assistance.
- promotes general well-being and health.

5. Mental Training Methods:

- Visualization: Use strategies for mental visualization to improve performance and attention.
- Mindfulness Practices: To reduce stress and increase mental resilience, use mindfulness or meditation practices.

- improves focus and mental clarity while working on exercises.
- promotes mental health in general.

6. Differential Training Approaches:

- Alternative workouts: To challenge and stimulate different muscle groups, combine workouts from several disciplines.
- Diverse Cardiovascular Exercises: To provide cardiovascular variation, use exercises like swimming, rowing, or cycling.

- avoids training boredom and possible plateaus.
- builds a flexible and all-encompassing foundation for fitness.

7. Weeks of Periodization and Deloading:

- Periodization: Divide your workouts into discrete stages and modify the volume and intensity.
- Deload Weeks: To promote recuperation and guard against overtraining, schedule weeks of reduced training intensity.

- improves long-term development by averting injuries and exhaustion.
- encourages long-term training consistency.

8. Consulting with Experts in Fitness:

- Fitness Evaluation: To find areas for development and get tailored advice, get expert evaluations.
- Professional Advice: To customize your program to meet your specific requirements, speak with nutritionists, physical therapists, or trainers.

- gives specific guidance on how to maximize your training.
- makes sure complementing components are integrated safely and effectively.

Through the deliberate integration of these components into your current training regimen, you establish a comprehensive and flexible strategy that optimizes your chances of success. By customizing these elements to meet your unique requirements and achieve your objectives, you can create a complete training program that surpasses simple exercises and unlocks new potential for performance and well-being.

Chapter 5

PERFORMANCE OPTIMIZATION

Maximizing Strength, Flexibility, and Coordination

Reaching optimal physical performance requires a well-rounded and all-encompassing strategy that tackles coordination, strength, and flexibility in concert. You may improve your athletic performance, lower your chance of injury, and realize the full potential of your body by using specific tactics for each component. For an integrated and comprehensive approach, here's how to enhance strength, flexibility, and coordination:

1. Strengthening Up:

Put into practice:

- Progressive Resistance Training: Include a systematic strength training regimen that works for various muscle groups in a step-by-step manner.
- Compound Movements: To work numerous muscular groups at once, concentrate on compound movements like bench presses, deadlifts, and squats.
- Periodization: To encourage ongoing adaptation, divide your strength training into periods with differing volumes and intensities.

Advantages:

- enhances total strength and adds lean muscular mass.
- improves the functionality of movement patterns and joint stability.
- strengthens connective tissues, assisting in the avoidance of injuries.

2. Adaptability Improvement:

- Dynamic Stretching: To increase flexibility while preserving muscular activation, make dynamic stretching a priority before working out.
- Static Stretching: To lengthen muscles and encourage relaxation, use static stretches during cool-down activities.

+ Incorporate Proprioceptive Neuromuscular Facilitation (PNF) stretching methods to get a higher level of muscle activation.

Advantages:
+ increases the range of motion while lowering the chance of injury.
+ increases joint flexibility and muscular elasticity.
+ encourages improved alignment and posture.

3. Development of Motor Skills and Coordination:

Participate:
+ Functional Movements: To enhance functional coordination, use workouts that resemble everyday tasks.
+ Balance Training: To improve proprioception, use balance exercises including single-leg stands and stability ball activities.
+ Agility training: To increase general responsiveness, combine agility training with fast, coordinated movements.

Advantages:
+ improves motor abilities and neuromuscular coordination.
+ increases dynamic stability and response time.
+ encourages the smooth fusion of suppleness and strength in motion.

4. Coordinated Training Guidelines:

Take up:
+ Cross-training: Take part in exercises like yoga, pilates, or functional fitness programs that combine coordination, strength, and flexibility.
+ Circuit Training: Design circuits with a mix of coordination problems, flexibility activities, and strength training.
+ Sport-Specific Training: Design exercises with the demands of your particular sport or activity in mind, putting special emphasis on the strength, flexibility, and coordination components that are needed.

Advantages:
+ guarantees that physical features grow in a well-rounded manner.
+ increases resilience and adaptation in a variety of physical activities.
+ enhances overall athleticism by tackling many issues at once.

5. Extensive Preparation and Detoxification:

- Dynamic Warm-Up: Give special attention to dynamic exercises that increase joint mobility and blood flow while getting the body ready for the next session.
- Recovering Actively Cool-down: To promote muscular healing and flexibility, including low-intensity activities and stretching in this period.

Advantages:
- reduces the chance of damage during exercise and maximizes the body's potential for performance.
- helps muscles recuperate after exercise by easing pain and stiffness.

6. Practices for the Mind-Body Connection:

- Exercises that emphasize the mind-body connection and foster awareness of movement and body alignment are referred to as mindful movement.
- Breathwork: To improve focus and relaxation, use regulated breathing methods while doing activities.
- Visualization: To improve coordination and reinforce appropriate movement patterns, use mental images.

Advantages:
- improves hand-eye coordination and motor control.
- eases tension and encourages an optimistic outlook during exercise.
- encourages a closer connection between the mind and body.

7. Regular Observation and Modification:

Put into practice:
- Regular Evaluations: Evaluate your coordination, strength, and flexibility regularly to monitor your development and pinpoint areas that need work.
- workout Intensity Adjustment: Adapt the volume and intensity of your workout to your current fitness level and objectives.
- Utilize responsive programming to modify your exercise regimen in response to your body's signals, resulting in a well-rounded and long-lasting strategy.

Advantages:
- encourages ongoing development and guards against plateaus.
- lowers the possibility of burnout and overtraining.
- makes it possible to make precise changes to remedy certain flaws.

By incorporating these techniques into your training regimen, you may enhance your strength, flexibility, and coordination by developing a comprehensive and linked strategy. This all-encompassing strategy enhances lifespan in physical endeavors as well as general well-being and athletic performance

How Fascia Supports Muscle Function

The dynamic and complex network of connective tissues known as the fascial system is essential to the maintenance and regulation of muscle function. Fascia is an active, responsive tissue that goes much beyond passive wrapping to support the health of muscles, the effectiveness of movements, and the general biomechanical integrity of the body. Now let's see how fascia facilitates muscle function:

1. Support and Integrity of Structure:

- Muscle Encapsulation: A sheath of fascia surrounds each muscle, providing protection and structural support.
- Muscles are divided into discrete compartments by a process called compartmentalization, which helps to organize and coordinate different muscle groups.

Effect:

- makes ensuring the body's muscles are stable and positioned correctly.
- allows for the effective transfer of force during motion.

2. Distribution and Transmission of Force:

- Myofascial Chains: Connected fascia chains that connect muscles and distribute force throughout the body.
- Tensional forces equally distribute load and tension across the fascial network according to the tensegrity (tensional integrity) concept.

Effect:

- allows muscle forces to be transferred smoothly, improving movement coordination.
- lessens the targeted strain on certain muscles, which improves overall performance.

3. Combined Mobility and Stabilization:

- Together with joint capsules, it integrates to provide support and stability.
- Facial Slings: By using slings or bands to connect muscles and joints, facial slings help promote coordinated movement patterns.

Effect:
- increases joint stability and lowers the chance of injury.
- promotes total mobility by making joint motions more fluid and controlled.

4. Elasticity of Tissue and Hydration:
- Ground material: Consists of a gel-like ground material that preserves fascial flexibility when adequately hydrated.
- Hydration inhibits the formation of adhesions and limitations in the fascial layers.

Effect:
- assures ideal tissue elasticity, enabling muscles to move over their whole range of motion.
- encourages receptive and dynamic movement patterns.

5. Proprioception and Sensory Feedback:
- Mechanoreceptors: Mechanoreceptors that provide sensory feedback are housed inside the fascial matrix.
- Proprioceptive input: Provides the central nervous system with data on joint position, muscle length, and tension.

Effect:
- improves proprioception and bodily awareness.

6. Myofascial Release Facilitation: Enables precise and coordinated motions based on real-time input.

- Innate Elasticity: Returns elasticity and releases tension in response to myofascial release treatments.
- Facilitates smooth fascial gliding across layers, avoiding constriction.

Effect:

- lessens muscular discomfort and promotes muscle healing.
- improves the general flexibility and health of the muscles.

7. Flexibility and Reaction to Stress:

- Collagen Fiber Orientation: The direction of applied tension determines how the collagen fibers inside the fascia align.
- Dynamic Adaptation: Modifies its composition and structure in response to variations in load and movement patterns.

Effect:

- makes it easier to adjust to different workouts and physical activities.
- enhances the body's capacity to resist and adjust to outside influences.

Comprehending the important function of fascia in endorsing muscular performance offers discernment into the intricate structure of the musculoskeletal system. Through specific activities like myofascial release, hydration, and diversity in movement, people may improve overall movement quality, minimize the chance of injury, and maximize muscle function by fostering the health and resilience of fascia. The dynamic interaction between muscles and fascia emphasizes how important it is to address physical well-being holistically.

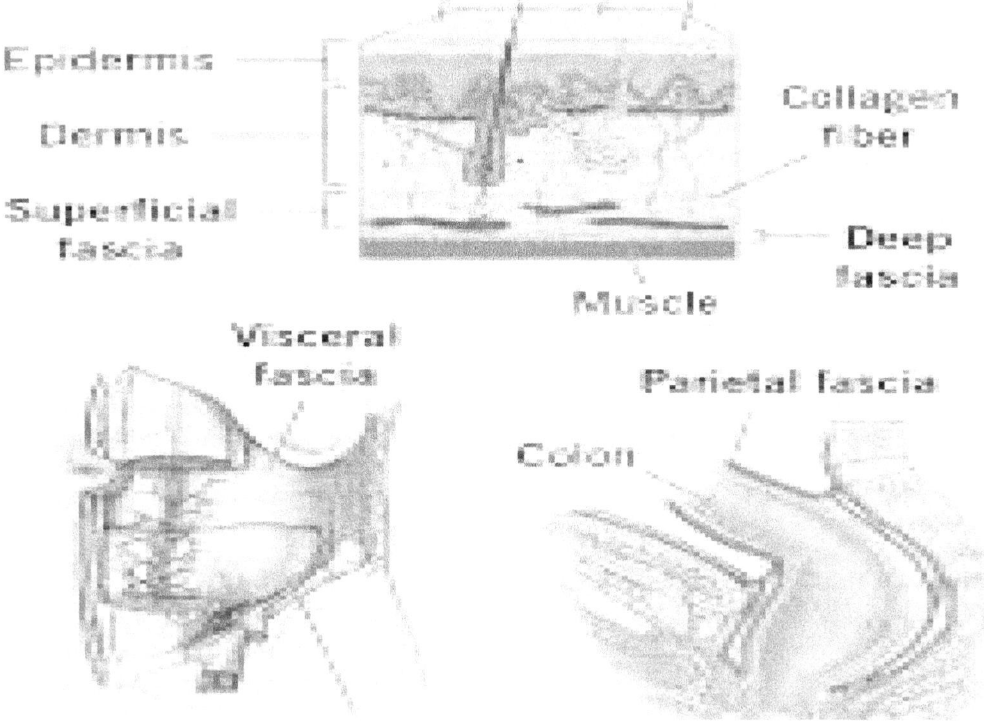

A deliberate emphasis on improving speed, agility, and power—essential elements that lead to success in a variety of sports and physical activities—is necessary to reach optimum athletic performance. Through the implementation of an all-encompassing training methodology that targets these components in concert, athletes may reach their maximum potential and demonstrate exceptional dynamic and explosive movement. Here's how you gradually improve your power, speed, and agility for the best possible athletic performance:

1. Acceleration Development:

- ➢ Sprint Training: To increase acceleration and peak speed, include quick bursts of sprints at maximum effort.
- ➢ Form exercises: Include particular exercises that concentrate on stride length, frequency, and running mechanics.
- ➢ Assisted and Overspeed Training: For resisted sprints, use resistance bands; for overspeed training, use downhill running.

Advantages:
- ➢ improves the frequency and efficiency of strides.
- ➢ improves neuromuscular adaptations for high-speed running and quick acceleration.

2. Instruction in Agility:

- ➢ Ladder exercises: Practice ladder exercises to enhance your coordination, footwork, and ability to shift directions quickly.
- ➢ Cone Drills: To practice quick direction changes and deceleration, set up agility courses using cones.
- ➢ Sport-unique Drills: To improve agility unique to your sport, mimic the motions needed in that particular activity.

Advantages:
- ➢ increases reactivity to direction adjustments and reaction speed.
- ➢ improves body control and proprioception during quick motions.

3. The Development of Power:

- ➢ Plyometric workouts: To build strength, include quick motions like medicine ball tosses, box jumps, and squat jumps.
- ➢ Olympic Weightlifting: To improve explosive strength, use Olympic lifts like snatches and cleans.
- ➢ Dynamic Strength Training: Do resistance exercises like jump squats and kettlebell swings with a focus on power and speed.

Advantages:
- ➢ speeds up the creation of force during explosive actions.
- ➢ enhances the capacity to produce power in the upper and lower limbs.

4. Combining Power, Agility, and Speed Drills:

- ➢ Circuit Training: Create circuits with a mix of power, agility, and speed workouts.
- ➢ Sport-Specific Exercises: Create exercises that smoothly include the power, speed, and agility elements specific to your sport.
- ➢ Reaction Training: Incorporate exercises that call for fast responses to aural or visual signals.

Advantages:
- ➢ improves the capacity to smoothly switch between power, agility, and speed movements.
- ➢ enhances total athleticism by integrating different aspects of physical performance.

5. Dynamic Mobility and Warm-Up:

- ➢ Joint Mobilization Exercises: Prepare the body for explosive activities by engaging in dynamic exercises that focus on major joints.
- ➢ Muscle Activation: Use modest resistance workouts and dynamic stretches to activate your muscles.
- ➢ Neuromuscular priming: Use nervous system-stimulating exercises to maximize output of power and speed.

Advantages:

- ➢ gets the body ready to exert itself.
- ➢ lowers the possibility of injuries brought on by forceful motions.

6. Training in Acceleration and Deceleration:

- ➢ Start Techniques: Work on quick beginnings to accelerate in sports-specific actions such as sprinting.
- ➢ Braking Drills: To increase dexterity and lower the chance of injury during quick stops, practice controlled deceleration methods.
- ➢ Exercises for Change of Pace: Include short bursts of varying intensity to improve your ability to accelerate and decelerate quickly.

Advantages:

- ➢ enhances the capacity to accelerate rapidly from a stop.
- ➢ improves stability and control while making abrupt stops and direction changes.

7. Training in Decision-Making and Reaction Time:

- ➢ Exercises in Agility Including Cognitive Elements: Combine agility activities with decision-making exercises that happen quickly.
- ➢ Both auditory and visual cues: To develop fast responses, use stimuli such as lights, music, or signals from your partner.
- ➢ Situations Specific to a Sport: Play scenarios that are similar to games and require fast decision-making.

Advantages:

- ➢ improves motor-cognitive coordination.
- ➢ enhances decision-making in high-speed scenarios on the field.

8. Recuperation Techniques:

- ➢ Dynamic and static stretching should be included in your post-training routine to promote flexibility and muscle healing.
- ➢ Rehabilitation Techniques: To lessen muscular discomfort, try compression treatment or a cold-water immersion.
- ➢ Sufficient Rest: To provide for the best possible recuperation, make sure you take enough time off in between intense training sessions.

Advantages:

helps muscles recuperate and lowers the possibility of overtraining.

encourages sustained sustainability in high-intensity exercise.

You may develop a comprehensive and focused training program that improves speed, agility, and power by using these principles. In addition to increasing athletic performance, this all-encompassing training approach lowers the chance of injury, increases general resilience, and develops dynamic and adaptive athleticism.

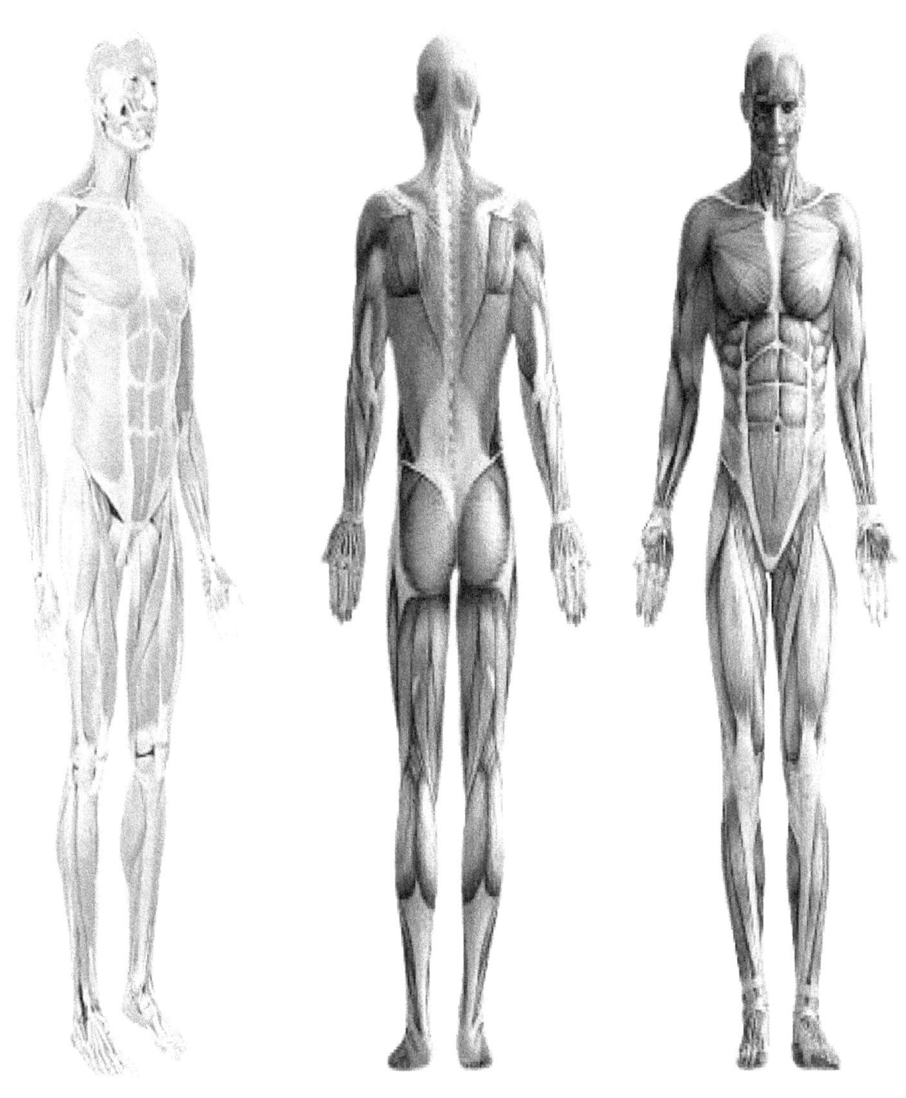

Chapter 6

INJURY PREVENTION AND REDUCTION

Injury prevention is essential for maintaining peak performance and long-term well-being in the world of sports and physical activities. A comprehensive strategy that includes biomechanical knowledge, strategic training methods, and recuperation techniques forms the basis for reducing the likelihood of injuries and encouraging a long-term athletic career.

1. Thorough Warm-up and Dynamic Stretching: It is crucial to start every training session with a dynamic stretching and warm-up regimen. This improves the range of motion and flexibility while also preparing the muscles and joints for the impending physical demands. A prepared body is less likely to suffer strains or sprains since it is better able to withstand force.

2. Strength and Conditioning Protocols: Programs with a structured approach to strength and conditioning are essential for preventing injuries. Achieving general biomechanical harmony involves targeting particular muscle groups, stabilizing joints, and treating muscular imbalances. Through the development of muscular strength, stamina, and joint stability, athletes build a strong foundation that protects against frequent injuries.

3. Functional Movement Assessment: Regularly doing functional movement evaluations helps to detect asymmetries and biomechanical inefficiencies that might put a person at risk for injury. By correcting these imbalances with focused workouts and treatments, movement patterns are improved, performance is maximized, and the risk of overuse injuries is reduced.

4. Activity-specific Training and Technique Improvement: By designing training plans that closely resemble the demands of a particular activity, players may acquire the abilities and fortitude needed to compete. Injury prevention is also greatly aided by honing tactics and using appropriate body mechanics during competition and training.

5. Periodization and Sufficient Recovery: It's essential to put into practice a well-organized periodization strategy that includes sufficient rest and recovery periods. Excessive exercise combined with little rest might make you tired, perform worse, and get hurt more easily. Rest periods enable the body to heal and adjust, lowering the possibility of overuse problems brought on by extended physical strain.

6. Cross-Training and Diverse Workouts: Mixing up your workouts and using cross-training exercises keeps things interesting and lowers your chance of repetitive strain injuries. Exercise exposes the body to a variety of stressors, fostering adaptation and resilience in general.

7. Nutritional Support and Hydration: The cornerstones of injury prevention are appropriate diet and hydration. Sufficient nutritional intake promotes tissue regeneration and repair, and ideal hydration preserves joint lubrication and normal physiological processes.

8. Frequent Monitoring and Screening: Early detection of possible problems is made possible by regular screenings in addition to frequent physical condition monitoring of athletes. Emerging problems may be addressed early on in training program modifications and interventions to prevent injury.

Injury prevention is, after all, a whole-person undertaking that happens off the training field. It represents a proactive and conscientious approach to sports activities, stressing the value of training, biomechanical awareness, and continuous improvement to support long-term performance and health. Athletes who prioritize injury prevention measures invest in a resilient and long-lasting athletic future in addition to protecting their existing skills.

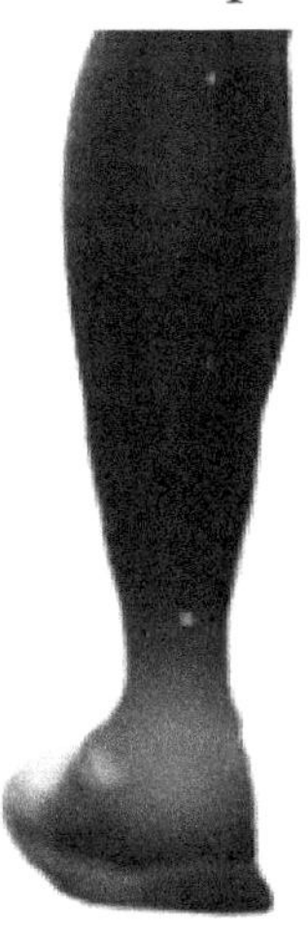
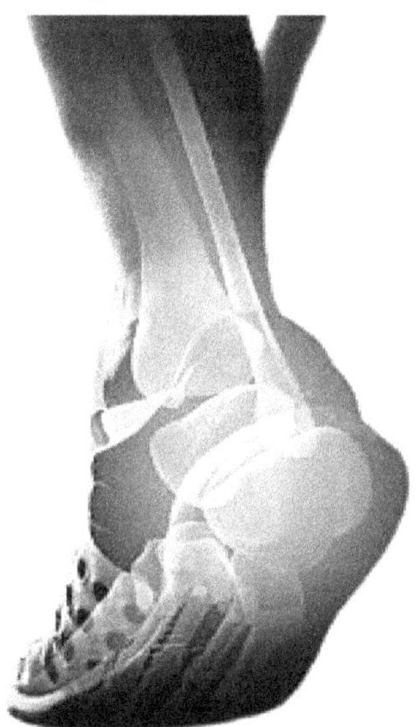

Identifying Imbalances and Restrictions

A sensitive awareness of imbalances and constraints that may obstruct optimum mobility is necessary to comprehend the complex interactions between the human body. Finding these limits and asymmetries is an essential first step in creating focused therapies, encouraging biomechanical balance, and enhancing general well-being.

1. Movement evaluations: The first step in identifying imbalances and limitations is to conduct thorough movement evaluations. In these evaluations, basic movement patterns are observed, and joint mobility, stability, and general coordination are examined. Finding departures from ideal movement patterns provides important information about possible problem locations.

2. Biomechanical Analysis: Applying methods and instruments for biomechanical analysis helps to improve our comprehension of imbalances. Assessing joint angles, muscle activation patterns, and gait analysis may be part of this. Through an exploration of the nuances of biomechanics, professionals may identify certain regions where constraints or asymmetries may impair effective movement.

3. Postural Evaluation: It's important to watch and examine someone's posture to spot any abnormalities that could be causing pain or a reduction in functioning. Muscle imbalances, joint constraints, and habitual behaviors may all contribute to poor posture, and correcting these problems is crucial to achieving ideal alignment again.

4. Range of Motion Evaluations: Determining the range of motion in different joints may assist in identifying limitations that can impede effective movement. Restricted ranges may be a sign of biomechanical barriers such as stiff joints, taut muscles, or others. To alleviate these restrictions, targeted flexibility exercises and joint mobilization methods might be used.

5. Functional Testing: Including functional tests that mimic activities pertinent to a person's sport or way of life offers a practical viewpoint on imbalances. Functional testing evaluates the body's ability to adjust to the demands of certain activities in addition to identifying limitations or shortcomings.

6. Symmetry Analysis: It's important to compare the symmetry of the left and right sides of the body. Differences in a side's strength, flexibility, or gait might point to imbalances that should be corrected. Resolving these imbalances encourages balance and lowers the possibility of overuse accidents.

7. Adaptability Variations: Disparities in muscle group flexibility may reveal abnormalities affecting joint mobility and general quality of movement. These disparities are addressed by using focused stretching regimens and flexibility exercises, which encourage a more balanced and fluid range of motion.

8. Functional History and Lifestyle Assessment: Understanding a person's prior injuries, routine activities, and lifestyle decisions provide important background information. Comprehending the role that lifestyle variables play in creating imbalances facilitates the customization of therapies to target particular issues and encourage long-lasting adjustments.

9. Constant Monitoring: Because the body is dynamic and adaptable, it is essential to conduct constant monitoring. Frequent reevaluation makes it possible to monitor development and spot new imbalances or limitations. A proactive and individualized approach to movement optimization is ensured by modifying treatments in response to continuing evaluations.

Through the methodical identification of imbalances and limits, coaches, practitioners, and people themselves may create focused methods for improvement. Resolving these issues improves performance, prevents injuries, and promotes general physical well-being in addition to improving movement quality. The path to ideal mobility starts with a deep understanding of the body's particular subtleties and a dedication to building resilience and balance.

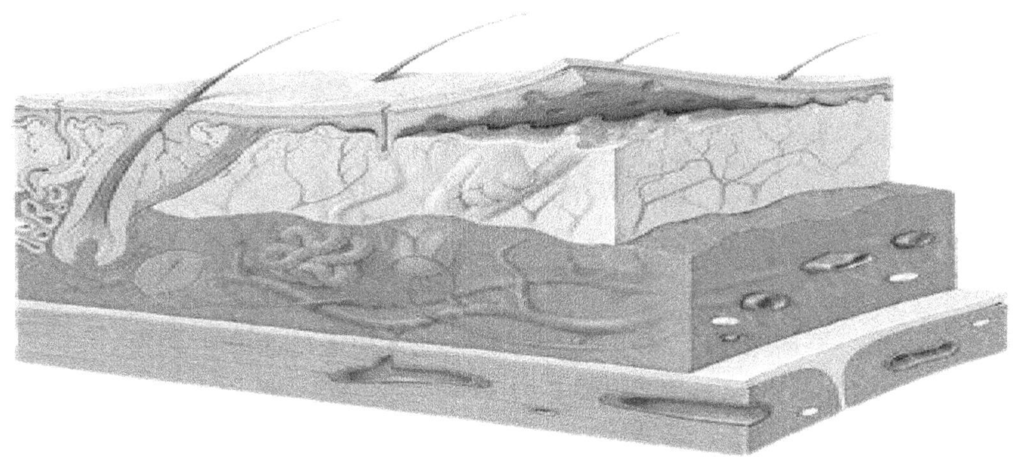

Sports activities provide the rush of physical accomplishment and competitiveness, but they also carry the danger of injury. Both athletes and fitness lovers must take a proactive and comprehensive approach to injury prevention. The risk of common sports injuries may be considerably decreased by people incorporating specific tactics into their training regimens and lifestyle choices.

1. Extensive Warm-up and Dynamic Stretching: It is essential to start each training session with an extensive warm-up and dynamic stretching regimen. Improving flexibility and range of motion gets the muscles, joints, and connective tissues ready for the impending physical demands. Strains, sprains, and other soft tissue injuries are less common in a body that has warmed up appropriately.

2. Stability and Firmness Training: Including strength and stability training in exercise routines helps increase the tensile strength of muscles and joints. Total biomechanical integrity is improved by concentrating on muscle imbalances, bolstering core stability, and treating weak regions. Consequently, this lessens the possibility of injuries brought on by inadequate joint stability and muscular support.

3. Emphasis on Correct Form and Technique: Performing exercises with correct form and technique is essential for preventing injuries. Stressing proper biomechanics avoids needless strain on joints and muscles and lowers the chance of overuse injuries whether lifting weights, doing agility exercises, or participating in sport-specific motions.

4. moderate Progression and Periodization: By combining planned periodization with moderate increases in training volume and intensity, the body can adjust gradually. Sudden increases in workload might raise the risk of injury and cause overtraining. Periodization, with its scheduled periods of rest and recuperation, reduces the chance of fatigue-related ailments while promoting sustained performance.

5. Training for Flexibility and Mobility: Retaining ideal joint mobility and flexibility is essential for preventing injuries. It is possible to avoid muscular imbalances and lower the risk of strains or tears during dynamic movements by regularly implementing mobility drills, static and dynamic stretching exercises, and both.

Ensuring sufficient rest and recuperation is essential for the body's capacity to mend and adjust. Weariness, decreased performance, and an elevated risk of injury might result from inadequate recuperation time. An efficient approach to preventing injuries must include rest days, healthy eating, and enough sleep.

7. Cross-Training and Variable Workouts: Overuse injuries may be avoided by varying workout regimens by including different exercise modalities and cross-training. Participating in diverse activities presents unique challenges to the body, hence mitigating the likelihood of recurring strain on certain muscles or joints that may arise from monotonous training.

8. Hydration and Nutrition: Maintaining healthy levels of both these nutrients is essential for preventing injuries. A healthy diet supplies vital nutrients for the health of muscles and connective tissues, and maintaining proper fluid levels promotes joint lubrication. Meeting dietary demands promotes healing and lowers the chance of injuries brought on by weariness.

9. Frequent Medical Exams and Screenings:

Regular screenings and check-ups for health problems may help find underlying conditions that might increase the risk of harm. Customized therapies to promote general well-being and reduce injury susceptibility may be made possible by addressing pre-existing conditions or risk factors.

10. Injury-Specific Rehabilitation: It is crucial to follow specific rehabilitation activities and see a specialist if you have ever had an injury. Reducing the chance of re-injury and promoting a complete and long-lasting recovery are achieved by addressing any remaining weaknesses and imbalances.

People may lay a strong foundation for their athletic endeavors by using this all-encompassing approach to injury avoidance. Preventive actions and a dedication to general physical fitness not only lower the likelihood of frequent sports injuries but also support sustained performance and long-term health.

Common musculoskeletal ailments that may interfere with physical activity and impair performance include strains, sprains, and tears. To ensure a thorough and long-lasting recovery, treating these injuries calls for a careful, multifaceted strategy that includes urgent treatment, rehabilitation, and preventative measures.

1. Immediate treatment and R.I.C.E Protocol: It's critical to provide timely and appropriate treatment after suffering a strain, sprain, or tear. The basic structure for first management is provided by the R.I.C.E. protocol, which stands for Rest, Ice, Compression, and Elevation. Compression offers support, elevating the injured region helps decrease inflammation, ice is used to lower swelling, and resting the area prevents more damage.

2. Professional treatment and Diagnosis: To precisely evaluate the degree of the damage, you must seek quick medical treatment. To ascertain the severity and best course of action, medical experts including physiotherapists and orthopedic specialists may do comprehensive exams, imaging investigations, and functional evaluations.

3. Physical therapy and rehabilitation exercises: Physical therapists often oversee structured rehabilitation programs, which are essential for both recovering functioning and averting further problems. Exercises designed specifically for the afflicted region improve and progressively restore mobility to the weakened muscles, ligaments, or tendons.

4. Progressive Loading and Gradual Return to Activity: A progressive loading strategy guarantees a safe and efficient return to activity as the wounded region recovers. Exercises that are progressively more difficult and intense aid in the restoration of stability, strength, and flexibility while lowering the chance of re-injury.

5. Manual Therapies and Modalities: Applying manual therapies may help relieve muscular tension, increase flexibility, and improve the general health of tissues. Examples of these therapies include massage, joint mobilization, and myofascial release. As adjuvants to aid in healing, modalities like electrical stimulation or ultrasound may also be used.

6. Addressing Biomechanical Problems: Long-term rehabilitation depends on identifying and resolving the underlying biomechanical problems that led to the injury. Through focused workouts and remedial techniques, this may include addressing muscle imbalances, enhancing joint stability, and honing movement patterns.

7. Psychological Support and Rehabilitation: Part of the healing process is realizing how the psychological effects of injuries might affect a person. Athletes might feel agitated, frustrated, or afraid of hurting themselves again. Psychological support—such as counseling or sports psychology interventions—assists people in overcoming these obstacles and cultivates an optimistic outlook on recovery.

8. Nutritional Support for Healing: The process of healing depends heavily on having an optimal diet. Sufficient consumption of protein aids in the repair of tissues, and vital nutrients such as vitamins and minerals enhance the general health of tissues. Working together with a nutritionist guarantees a comprehensive strategy to assist healing.

9. Injury Prevention techniques: It is critical to put injury prevention techniques into practice as soon as meaningful rehabilitative progress is made. To lower the likelihood of recurring strains, sprains, or rips, this entails consistent exercise, mobility work, and lifestyle adjustments.

10. A Gradual Comeback to Performance Enhancement and Sport:

For sustained performance, returning to sports or physical activities must be done gradually and methodically. To guarantee that the person is suitably conditioned and ready for the demands of their particular activity, coordination with coaches, trainers, and medical specialists is necessary.

Beyond emergency treatment, treating sprains, strains, and tears calls for a comprehensive, patient-centered approach. Individuals may reduce the likelihood of future musculoskeletal problems by developing resilience and healing from acute injury via the integration of complete rehabilitation procedures and addressing contributory variables. To achieve a full and long-lasting recovery, cooperation between medical experts, rehabilitation specialists, and the patients themselves is essential.

Chapter 7

RECOVERY AND TISSUE HEALTH

Post-Workout and Competition Recovery

Athlete performance is mostly dependent on their ability to recover from workouts and competitions effectively. This allows their bodies to recuperate quickly and be ready for new challenges. This all-encompassing recuperation procedure includes calculated steps that support energy restoration, fatigue management, and muscle regeneration to enhance general health and long-term sports performance.

1. Instant Cool-down and Stretching: Start the healing process right away with a quick cool-down. Reduce the level of physical activity gradually to facilitate the body's shift from a high-energy state to a resting one. Include static stretching to help release tension and increase muscular flexibility.

2. Hydration and Electrolyte Replenishment: Drinking enough water after working out vigorously or competing is essential for recuperation. Drink water to regain fluid balance, and think about electrolyte-containing drinks to replace vital minerals lost via perspiration.

3. Diet for Muscle Recovery: Following an exercise session, proper nutrition is essential for promoting muscle recovery. Muscle protein synthesis is improved and glycogen levels are replenished when a mix of carbs and protein is consumed in the first thirty to one hour after exercise. For the best possible recovery, include sources of complex carbs and lean protein.

4. Cryotherapy and Contrast Baths: Ice baths and contrast baths, which alternate between hot and cold water, are examples of cold treatments that may help lessen discomfort and inflammation in the muscles. By encouraging both vasoconstriction and vasodilation, these methods improve blood flow and hasten the excretion of metabolic waste.

5. Compression Garments: After a workout or competition, using compression garments might help minimize perceived discomfort and muscular edema. These clothes provide pressure, which promotes blood flow and keeps waste products from the metabolism from building up.

6. Active Recovery Exercises: As part of an active recovery regimen, doing low-intensity, aerobic exercises increases blood flow to the muscles, which helps eliminate waste and improves nutrition delivery. Swimming, cycling, and light running are a few types of efficient active rehabilitation workouts.

7. Massage and Foam Rolling: To relieve trigger points and tight muscles, self-myofascial release techniques combined with foam rolling are used. These methods improve general relaxation, lessen muscular stiffness, and increase flexibility.

8. Getting Enough Sleep: Getting enough sleep is essential to healing. The body goes through vital functions including muscle mending, growth hormone release, and general cellular renewal when you sleep. To maximize recuperation, aim for 7-9 hours of sleep without interruption.

9. Relaxation and Mental Recovery Techniques: Use relaxation and mental recovery techniques including deep breathing, mindfulness, and meditation. These methods encourage calmness, lessen tension, and foster optimism—all of which are essential for maintaining competitive sports performance.

10. Customized healing Plans: Understand that different people and sports have different healing requirements. Adjust recuperation schedules according to exercise length and intensity, personal fitness objectives, and particular sports ambitions. Reevaluate and modify recuperation plans regularly to keep up with changing training requirements.

Athletes may enhance long-term performance, minimize the danger of overtraining, and improve their body's resilience by using these post-workout and competition recovery measures. In addition to promoting physical well-being, a proactive and all-encompassing approach to rehabilitation promotes the mental and emotional components of athletic efforts, which adds to a well-rounded and long-lasting athletic journey.

After vigorous or unusual activity, muscular soreness, also known as delayed onset muscle soreness (DOMS), is a typical occurrence. While some pain is a normal reaction to exercise, athletes and fitness enthusiasts should try to minimize the amount of soreness and how long it lasts. Using focused techniques will help you properly manage and lessen your muscular discomfort.

Gradual Progress in Exercise Intensity: Sudden increases in volume or intensity of exercise are one of the main causes of soreness in the muscles. The probability and degree of soreness may be decreased by gradually increasing the intensity and length of exercises, which enables the muscles to adapt.

2. **Warm-up and Cool-down Routines:** Prioritize hard workouts with active warm-up movements. Improving blood flow and flexibility gets the muscles ready for action. Include a cool-down with static stretching after your workout to assist develop flexibility and help relax your muscles, which may help reduce discomfort.

3. **Sufficient Hydration and Diet:** Make sure you drink enough water before, during, and after physical activity. Muscle discomfort may worsen if you're dehydrated. To aid in muscle recovery and restore energy reserves, have a well-balanced post-exercise meal or snack that includes both protein and carbs.

4. **Ice and Cold Therapy:** Using cold packs or ice on aching muscles will assist in numbing pain receptors and decrease inflammation, which will relieve the affected area. For bigger muscular areas, ice baths or cold immersion may be beneficial, particularly after vigorous exercise.

5. **Active Recovery Workouts:** On rest days or as a component of an active recovery regimen, do mild, low-intensity workouts. Exercises that improve blood flow to the muscles, such as walking, swimming, or cycling, aid in the elimination of metabolic byproducts linked to pain.

6. **Massage and foam rolling:** Using foam rollers for self-myofascial release and massage treatment may help relieve pain and tightness in the muscles. By promoting blood circulation and dissolving adhesions, these methods facilitate healing.

7. Wearing Compression Garments: Compression garments may help to lessen felt discomfort and muscular edema. The pressure that these clothes provide helps blood flow and could make it easier for metabolic waste products to be expelled.

8. Good Posture and Ergonomics: By keeping your body in alignment throughout exercises and everyday tasks, you may reduce the amount of tension placed on your muscles and joints, which lowers your chance of experiencing pain. Make sure you are lifting weights or doing other workouts with good form and ergonomics.

9. Anti-Inflammatory Supplements: Some supplements have anti-inflammatory qualities, including turmeric and omega-3 fatty acids. By consuming these supplements, one's risk of inflammation and pain in the muscles may be decreased.

10. Sufficient Rest and Sleep: Good sleep is necessary for the repair of muscles. Aim for seven to nine hours of sound sleep every night. Muscles can heal and adapt when they get enough rest in between exercises, which lowers the risk of chronic pain.

11. Consistent Training: Stick to a regular workout schedule so that your body can adjust over time. Increased muscular discomfort during periods of inactivity might be attributed to irregular training routines.

12. Over-the-Counter Pain Relief: Advise caution while using over-the-counter pain medicines such as acetaminophen or ibuprofen to treat muscular discomfort. But, if discomfort continues, it's crucial to see a doctor rather than depending only on medicine.

By using these techniques in your routine, you may reduce the effects of soreness in your muscles, making exercise more pleasant and long-lasting. For optimal performance and long-term well-being, it's critical to pay attention to your body, modify training volume as needed, and take a holistic approach to recuperation.

Sustaining an active and dynamic lifestyle, avoiding accidents, and preserving maximum physical function all depend critically on the vitality of total tissue health. The functions of tissues in movement and stability are interrelated and include muscles, tendons, ligaments, and fascia. Putting methods into practice to improve tissue health benefits not only short-term resilience and performance but also long-term well-being.

1. Proper Hydration: Water is essential for tissue health and cellular activity. Maintaining proper hydration promotes nutrition transit, lubricates joints, and speeds up cellular processes necessary for tissue healing. Staying hydrated is essential for the general health of your tissues.

2. Balanced Nutrition: For tissue health, a diet rich in nutrients and well-rounded is essential. Make sure you consume enough protein to aid in muscle regeneration, foods high in collagen to strengthen connective tissue, and a range of vitamins and minerals to enhance general tissue resilience. Foods high in antioxidants protect tissues from oxidative damage and lengthen their lifespan.

3. Frequent Physical Activity: Getting regular exercise increases blood flow, which nourishes and oxygenates all of the body's tissues. Exercise also promotes the synthesis of collagen, which is essential for the strength and flexibility of connective tissues.

4. Flexibility and Mobility Training: Consistently incorporating mobility and flexibility exercises improves the pliability of connective tissues and muscles. Stretching exercises increase the range of motion in joints, lessen stiffness, and improve the suppleness of tissues generally.

5. Strength Training: The development and maintenance of muscular mass depend heavily on resistance training. Robust muscles enhance tissue robustness overall, stabilize joints, and lower the chance of injury. Additionally, progressive resistance training increases collagen production, which improves the health of ligaments and tendons.

6. Sufficient Sleep and Recuperation: Restorative sleep is essential for tissue growth and repair. Growth hormone is released by the body when you sleep, which aids in the healing of muscles and tissues. Make sure you get enough sleep and recuperation to support the resilience and general health of your tissues.

7. Massage and Soft Tissue Therapies: Myofascial release and other regular massage techniques help to remove tension, adhesions, and knots in the muscles. These methods increase tissue pliability generally, release tense muscles, and increase blood circulation.

8. Supplementing with hyaluronic acid: Hyaluronic acid is a naturally occurring substance that helps lubricate joints and hydrate skin. Supplementation may sometimes help maintain the health of all tissues, especially in those who have dry skin or joint pain.

9. Posture Awareness: Reducing tissue tension requires maintaining good posture. Joint strain and muscular imbalances may be caused by poor posture. To support tissue alignment, regularly evaluate your posture throughout everyday tasks and during exercise.

10. Active Recovery and Gentle Movement: Activate your body to increase blood flow and aid in the elimination of waste products from metabolism. Without putting undue pressure on the tissues, gentle exercises like yoga, swimming, or walking may promote general tissue health.

11. Regular Health Check-ups: Regular screenings and check-ups enable the early identification of any problems impacting tissue health. Proactively addressing underlying health issues promotes total tissue well-being.

12. Stress Management: By increasing inflammation and obstructing healing processes, chronic stress may have a detrimental effect on tissue health. To enhance general tissue resilience, use stress-reduction strategies like mindfulness, meditation, or deep breathing.

A proactive and comprehensive strategy that incorporates workout routines, conscious self-care, and lifestyle choices is necessary to cultivate total tissue health. Making your body's foundation a priority supports both long-term health and resilience in addition to providing instant comfort and functionality.

Conclusion

I feel incredibly empowered and enlightened as we close the pages of this extensive guide, "Fascia Unleashed: Optimize Performance and Prevent Injuries with this Cutting-Edge Therapy," after this groundbreaking investigation into the world of fascia and the groundbreaking therapy it inspired. This journey has been more than just the discovery of a treatment strategy; it has been an invitation to comprehend, accept, and maximize the complex network that is the fascial system of our bodies.

This book is based on the idea that our bodies are wonderfully built and that we may achieve unmatched physical well-being by discovering the secrets hidden in our connective tissues. "Unleash the Power of Fascia" goes beyond the bounds of traditional methods to sports, rehabilitation, and general health to represent not just a treatment but a paradigm change in how we see and care for our bodies.

We studied the intriguing architecture of the fascial system, which links muscles, organs, and tissues and affects all aspects of movement and stability, to achieve optimum well-being. We investigated the deep connections that fascia forms throughout the body, comprehending how it affects flexibility, movement patterns, and overall physical performance.

"Unleash the Power of Fascia" was not created at random; rather, it was the result of a strong grasp of biomechanics, a dedication to scientific integrity, and a strong desire to maximize human potential. Our investigation, which covers everything from the beginnings and growth of this ground-breaking treatment to the changing field of biomechanics, has been grounded in evidence-based procedures to guarantee that you, the reader, are armed with the most recent knowledge and methods.

The methods in this book are not workouts; rather, they open doors to a whole new level of physical empowerment. Including these sessions in your practice is an invitation to take ownership of your fascial health and to set out on a path of self-awareness, resiliency, and steadfast vitality.

Our commitment to your health goes beyond what is mentioned. The comprehensive framework we have offered, including everything from anatomy lectures to tactics and a comprehensive strategy, is more than just a manual; it is an indication of our dedication to your success. "Fascia Unleashed" is a complete resource created by rigorous scientific research and verified by athletes, fitness professionals, and therapists. It is meant to change and adapt with you over time, giving you access to the most current and efficient procedures for your journey.

As you integrate these life-changing activities, keep in mind that this is a lifetime choice, a dedication to the continuous improvement of your physical well-being and, therefore, your overall quality of life. The holistic approach that is being promoted here is based on the notion that genuine well-being is a combination of mental, emotional, and physical health. It is not a fad.

Finally, let this be the beginning of a life that is enhanced by realizing and releasing the power that is inside your fascia, not its end. May the ideas and methods presented in these pages act as a spark for a lifetime of improved productivity, less chance of injury, and continued physical vigor.

Remember that the power of fascia is a reality that is simply waiting to be experienced as you go out on the road that lies ahead. Accept this as fact, live it, and let your fascia's untapped potential serve as your road map to an extraordinary future filled with unwavering vitality and well-being.

Appendix

SELF-ASSESSMENT TOOLS

HOW TO USE

- Complete the self-assessment regularly (e.g., every two weeks) to track changes over time.
- Compare current measurements and perceptions with initial baseline data.
- Use the worksheet as a tool for goal setting and adjusting your "Fascia Unleashed" routine.

SELF-ASSESSMENT WORKSHEET

PERSONAL INFORMATION: **NAME:** _______________ **DATE:** _________ **FITNESS LEVEL:** [B] [I] [A]

Section 1: Baseline Measurements

1. Range of Motion (ROM):
   - Record baseline measurements for key joints and movements (e.g., shoulder flexion, hip extension, spinal rotation).
   - Note any areas of stiffness or limitations.
2. Flexibility Assessment:
   - Perform basic flexibility tests (e.g., toe touch, hamstring stretch, quad stretch).
   - Rate your flexibility on a scale from 1 to 10 for each tested area.
3. Strength and Endurance:
   - Identify specific muscle groups targeted by "Fascia Unleashed."
   - Perform strength tests (e.g., plank, wall sit) and record your performance.

Section 2: Movement Patterns

1. Functional Movement Assessment:
2. Evaluate fundamental movement patterns (e.g., squat, lunge, push-up).
3. Identify any compensations, imbalances, or discomfort during movements.

Section 3: Therapy Integration

1. Frequency of Therapy Sessions:
2. Track how often you incorporate "Fascia Unleashed" therapy into your routine (e.g., sessions per week).
3. Perceived Benefits:
4. Rate your perceived benefits after each therapy session (e.g., improved flexibility, reduced muscle tension, enhanced mobility).

Section 4: Lifestyle and Well-being

1. Sleep Quality:
2. Rate the quality of your sleep on a scale from 1 to 10.
3. Note any changes in sleep patterns or improvements.
4. Stress Levels:
5. Assess your stress levels using a Likert scale.
6. Reflect on any stress reduction observed since starting the therapy.

Section 5: Overall Reflection

1. Overall Progress:
2. Reflect on your overall progress since starting "Fascia Unleashed."
3. Highlight specific achievements, challenges, or changes you've noticed.
4. Goals and Adjustments:
5. Define short-term and long-term goals related to your fascial health.
6. Identify any adjustments or modifications needed in your approach.

Section 6: Additional Notes

1. Notes and Observations:
2. Use this space for additional notes, observations, or any specific feedback.
3. Document any questions or concerns for future reference.

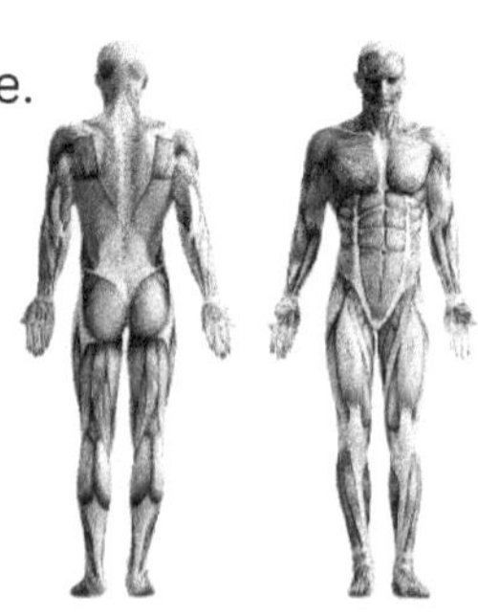